# Remi's Journey

## Tails of Love, Joy, and Hope

**JOHN V. RINALDO**

*Rinaldo & Partners Publishing*

# COPYRIGHTS

This work, including all text, characters, plotlines, and other original content, is the exclusive intellectual property of Rinaldo Partners and its author, John V. Rinaldo. No part of this work may be reproduced, distributed, or transmitted in any form or by any means, including photocopying, recording, or other electronic or mechanical methods, without the prior written permission of the copyright holder, except in the case of brief quotations embodied in critical reviews and certain other noncommercial uses permitted by copyright law.

Unauthorized reproduction or distribution of this work, whether in whole or in part, constitutes copyright infringement and may be subject to legal action and civil penalties. Any unauthorized use of the characters, storyline, or other elements of this work is strictly prohibited.

For permissions requests or other inquiries, please contact:

Rinaldo & Partners Publishing
Email: rinaldo@rinaldopartners.com
ISBN: 9798340049377
Website: Rinaldopartners.com
Cover design by Rinaldo & Partners Publishing

Protecting the integrity of this intellectual property is of utmost importance to Rinaldo Partners and John V. Rinaldo. Your respect for their creative work is greatly appreciated.

# DEDICATION

To my loved ones and, of course, to Remi—yes, Remi is a real dog, and I've come to love him as one of my own. The stories of Remi, the Rat Pack, and Izzy are based on true encounters that reflect the joy, companionship, and sometimes the mischief we share with our furry friends. Remi, with his boundless energy and heart, inspired me to write this book. As we've trained together each day, his obedience has greatly improved, but more than that, our bond has deepened. He's grown into a support dog, not only in title but in spirit.

The people in this book are real too—people who love their dogs and cherish them like family. They know, as I do, that dogs provide so much more than companionship—they offer unconditional love, loyalty, and a sense of peace that fills your heart. I have grown to admire their passion for animal welfare and appreciate their efforts to protect and advocate for animals, especially those who cannot speak for themselves.

I want to thank Remi's adopted mother for allowing me to be a part of Remi's life. Sometimes, we all need a sense of purpose and support, and often we don't even realize it until it finds us. Remi has filled that role in my life. And through this experience, I've gained a new understanding of the struggles and triumphs of adoption, not just for humans but for our pets as well. I also want to acknowledge and support those who fight tirelessly to stop animal cruelty and save mistreated pets. Your work to rescue and protect animals from cruel owners and harmful breeding practices is vital, and your efforts are deeply appreciated.

This book is dedicated to those who are about to adopt a dog. I hope Remi's story helps you understand the stress, emotions, and adjustments that a new dog may experience as they transition into their forever home. It's a journey for both you and your new furry friend, filled with challenges, but also incredible moments of joy and connection. I hope these stories offer comfort, patience, and a deeper understanding of the bond you're about to create.

To those who already love and care for their animals—you know how powerful that bond can be. May this book serve as a reminder to cherish every moment with your four-legged family members, for they give us more than we sometimes realize.

And finally, to all the animal advocates out there fighting every day to end cruelty and mistreatment, especially in harmful breeding kennels—thank you for your dedication. Without your compassion and hard work, the plight of these animals might go unnoticed. You are their voice, and you make a difference.

To my loved ones and to Remi—thank you for inspiring me to write this story. You've filled my life with love and joy, and I hope these stories bring that same warmth to everyone who reads them.

~ John Rinaldo

# CONTENTS

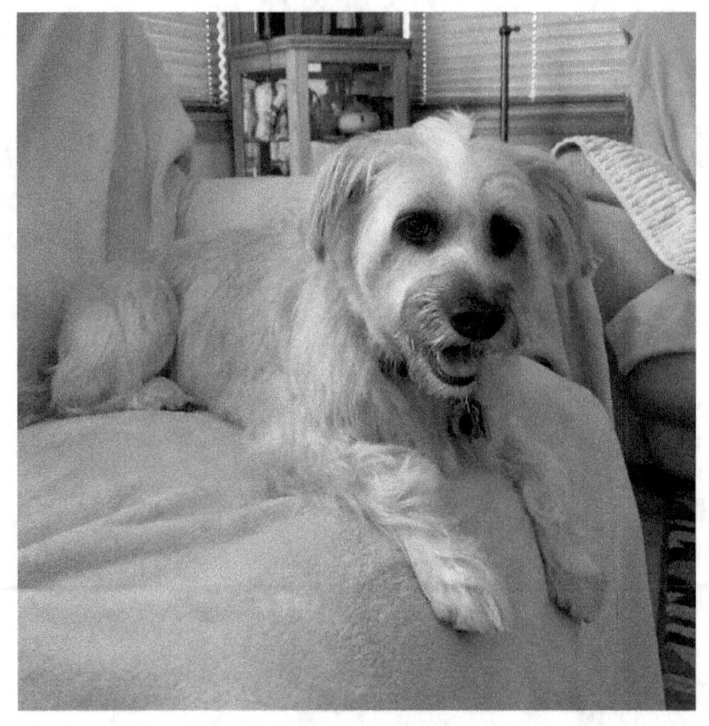

REMINGTON "REMI"

*"Money can buy you a fine dog,*
*but only love can make him wag his tail."*

– Kinky Friedman

# ACKNOWLEDGMENTS

Hello, friends! My name is Remington, but you can call me Remi. Yes, I'm a dog—just in case you hadn't guessed—and I have a very important job. It's my mission to remind my humans (and now you too!) that life is an adventure meant to be enjoyed, not a race to the finish line.

This book is my story, told from my perspective, about all the exciting places we explore, the challenges we face, and the lessons I teach my humans along the way. Whether we're on a simple walk in the park or experiencing life's bigger, more complicated moments, I'm always there to remind them that every step of the journey is worth savoring.

From learning new tricks with Dad to quiet evenings with Mom, and playdates with my brother Colt, Tigger, and Gus, every day holds something special. And let's not forget Daisy and the two cats who like to keep me on my paws! Life has been an incredible adventure with them, and it's been my joy to be their guide, reminding them to live in the moment.

To my family—Mom, Dad, Uncle Mike, Auntie Donna, Colt, Tigger, Gus, Daisy, and yes, even the two cats—you've filled my life with love and joy. Thank you for making this journey one I'll never forget. My days wouldn't be the same without you.

To you, my readers, I hope my tail... I mean, tale... brings a little wag to your life. Whether you're human or a fellow dog, always remember that we're all in this together. So, keep sniffing out the good things in life, embrace every moment, and never forget to enjoy the ride.

Thank you for joining me on this adventure. I can't wait to share more stories with you in the future!

Woof!

~ Remi

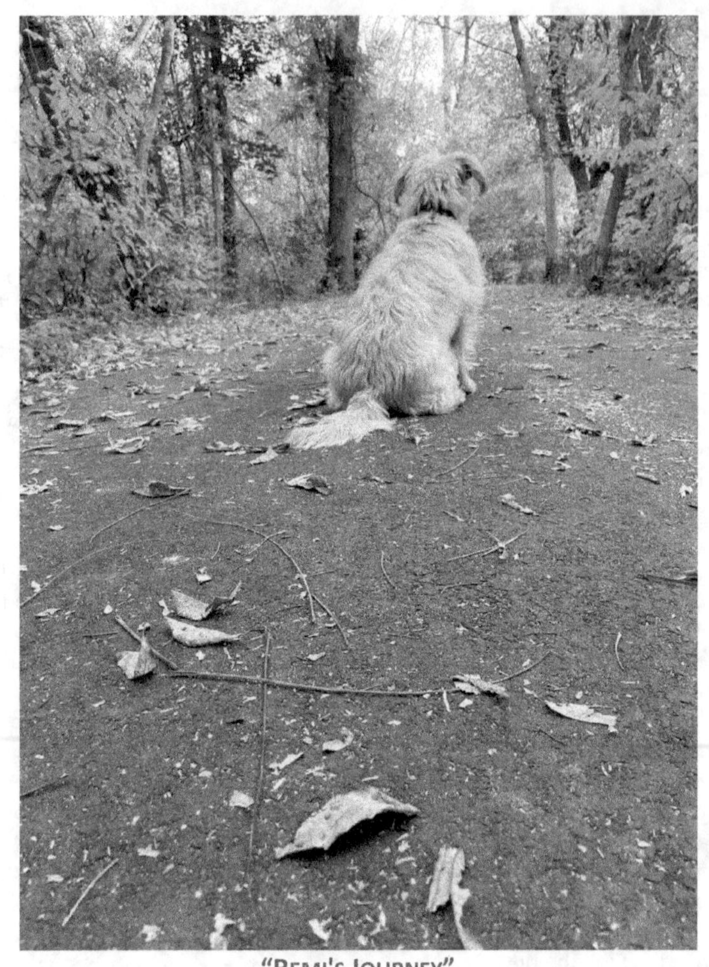



*"A dog wags its tail with its heart."*

– Martin Buxbaum

# INTRODUCTION
### *REMI, OUR LITTLE RAY OF SUNSHINE*

When Remi came into our lives, we never imagined how much one little dog could change everything. Remington, or "Remi" as we call him, is the newest and most joyful member of our family. While we're not entirely sure of his breed, we suspect that Cairn Terrier blood runs through his veins. With his scruffy coat, sparkling eyes, and an irresistible charm, Remi quickly became our beacon of light, a ray of sunshine that brightened the stormy seas of life.

From the moment we brought him home, we knew Remi was special. There was a calmness about him, a quiet but undeniable presence that immediately put us at ease. Life has a way of piling on worries and stress, creating heavy, unseen burdens that sometimes feel too much to bear. But with Remi around, it was as if that weight lifted, even if just for a moment. His wagging tail and excited bark greeted us every morning, reminding us that each day was a new beginning—a fresh start.

Remi's role as a support dog goes far beyond simple companionship. His true purpose is to help us, his human family, navigate the emotional ups and downs of life. Whenever the world feels like it's spinning too fast, or we're drowning in a sea of tasks and responsibilities, Remi is there to ground us. He has a unique ability to remind us that life isn't about racing to the finish line but about savoring each moment, one step at a time.

At first, Remi's adventures were simple—just walks around the neighborhood. He'd sniff the ground curiously, his tail wagging as if every scent told a story only, he could understand. For Remi, every moment was fresh and exciting—a chance to explore, feel, and truly be alive. Watching him, we began to realize how much of life we'd been missing. The beauty of a blooming flower, the warmth of the sun on our skin, the laughter of children playing in the park— these were things we had taken for granted. But not Remi. He embraced each moment with boundless enthusiasm.

Our little neighborhood walks soon turned into bigger adventures. We started taking Remi on nature hikes, where he'd bound up rocky trails with fearless energy, encouraging us to keep going, even when our legs grew tired. He'd pause every so often to look back, his eyes saying, "Come on, we can do this together." And somehow, we always could. We could climb those hills, cross those streams, and overcome our inner battles.

Remi's presence has taught us the importance of living in the present. His unconditional love and loyalty serve as constant reminders that there is beauty in simplicity. Whether it's cuddling on the couch after a long day, watching the sun set together, or simply enjoying a quiet moment in the garden, Remi brings us back to what truly matters: love, peace, and togetherness.

As we continue to explore life with Remi by our side, we hope his story brings a bit of light into yours. If you ever find yourself feeling lost, overwhelmed, or unsure of your next steps, remember the lessons we've learned from Remi: stay grounded, savor the journey, and most importantly, hold on to hope. After all, life is not about who finishes first; it's about cherishing each step along the way.

# CHAPTER 1
## *A NEW BEGINNING*

Before I became a support dog, my journey began in a small, cozy foster home. I was born in November 2021, during a time when the world was still healing from the chaos of the COVID-19 pandemic. The outside world felt uncertain, but inside our little bubble, everything was warm, safe, and filled with simple joys. My mother had given birth to seven of us—four brothers and three sisters. We were a tight-knit group, always exploring the limited space around us, though we knew nothing of the world beyond.

Our foster home was comforting, but deep down, we knew it wasn't forever. There were too many of us for one home to handle, and with the crisp fall air came the unmistakable scent of change. As winter approached, our mother would share stories of humans getting ready for something they called *"Thanksgiving,"* a time when families come together to celebrate. It sounded lovely, but as puppies, we only sensed that something big was coming—something beyond our understanding, a shift that would change our lives forever.

As I grew older, I came to appreciate the meaning of *"holidays,"* but in the beginning, I didn't like them at all. They were a reminder of when I was adopted, and holidays became a painful reminder of everything I had lost. But that's a story for another time.

One day, I overheard our foster parents talking about finding us new homes. They had posted on Facebook, searching for families who might want to adopt a puppy. I didn't quite understand what *"adoption"* meant, but I sensed it was something important. My mother, with her ever-calming presence, assured us, *"You are all special, and no matter where you go, I will always love you."* She was doing her best to comfort us, but I could feel the sadness in her voice.

Our birth was unexpected, as my mother was older and wasn't supposed to have more puppies—this was her second litter. She often talked about her first litter, though she had lost touch with them. I wondered if she would talk about us the same way when we were gone. The thought of never seeing my siblings or my mother again weighed heavily on my heart. I found a quiet corner to lie down, lost in thought about what my future would hold. Would I ever feel that warmth and safety again?

As I lay there, feeling confused and anxious, my older brother came and sat beside me. *"What's on your mind?"* he asked.

*"I'm scared,"* I admitted. *"I don't know what's going to happen. What if we never see each other or Mom again?"*

He paused, then said something that stayed with me: *"You can't live in the past or the future. You must live for now. Make the most of the present, little brother. That's where you'll find purpose."*

I tapped him on the back with my paw. *"Thank you,"* I said, feeling a bit lighter. Maybe change wasn't all bad.

The very next day, three human ladies came to visit. They seemed excited, their voices full of warmth and hope. As they looked at us, I could sense that they weren't just looking for any dog—they were searching for the right one. While my brothers and sisters were busy darting around, trying to get attention, I stayed back, letting my eyes do the work. I had always been told that my eyes had a way of speaking directly to the heart, and I hoped they would do the same for these humans.

Some say I have the spirit of a Cairn Terrier, and while I don't know for sure what I am, I knew I had the heart of a warrior—a heart full of love and loyalty, ready to serve and protect. The ladies were drawn to me, likely because of my scruffy coat and gentle gaze. But there was a problem—one of my brothers looked exactly like me.

I watched as the ladies debated, trying to figure out which one of us to choose. My heart pounded in my chest, hoping they would see that I was the one for them. After a few moments, the older woman pointed to my brother and said, *"I'll take this one."* My heart sank. Had I lost my chance?

But just as I was about to give up hope, the younger lady kneel down and looked straight into my eyes. She smiled warmly and said, *"I'm going to call my dog Remington—Remi for short."* My heart soared. She had chosen me! In that moment, I knew I was going home.

It turns out, I wasn't going alone. My older brother was coming too. The transition felt less scary knowing I had him by my side. We were leaving behind the only home we had ever known, but we were doing it together. As we said our goodbyes to our birth mother and siblings, my mother's words echoed in my mind: *"Take care of each other. You're all you have now, and remember, I will always love you."* Her words wrapped around me like a comforting blanket, and though it was hard to leave, I knew this was the start of something new and beautiful.

The older lady named my older brother Colt, a strong name for a strong pup. Having him with me made everything feel a little easier. Together, we embarked on this new adventure, heading toward a life full of love, joy, and purpose. We didn't know what was waiting for us, but I could feel it deep inside—this was where we were meant to be.

As the car pulled away from our foster home, the world outside felt both unfamiliar and full of promise. I caught a glimpse of my older brother beside me, and we exchanged a look that said, *"We've got this."* We were stepping into a new chapter, and although the future was unknown, I wasn't afraid anymore. I had Colt, and we had each other.

This was the beginning of a new life—a new family, a new home, and a new purpose. I didn't know it at the time, but this was the first step on my journey to becoming a support dog. It wasn't going to be easy, but I was ready to face whatever came my way.

And as the car drove on, I couldn't help but feel a mix of excitement and sadness. This was the last time Colt, and I would ever see our birth mother and siblings. The finality of it hit me, but I realized that change wasn't something to fear; it was something to embrace. The future was wide open, and I was ready to step into it, one paw at a time.

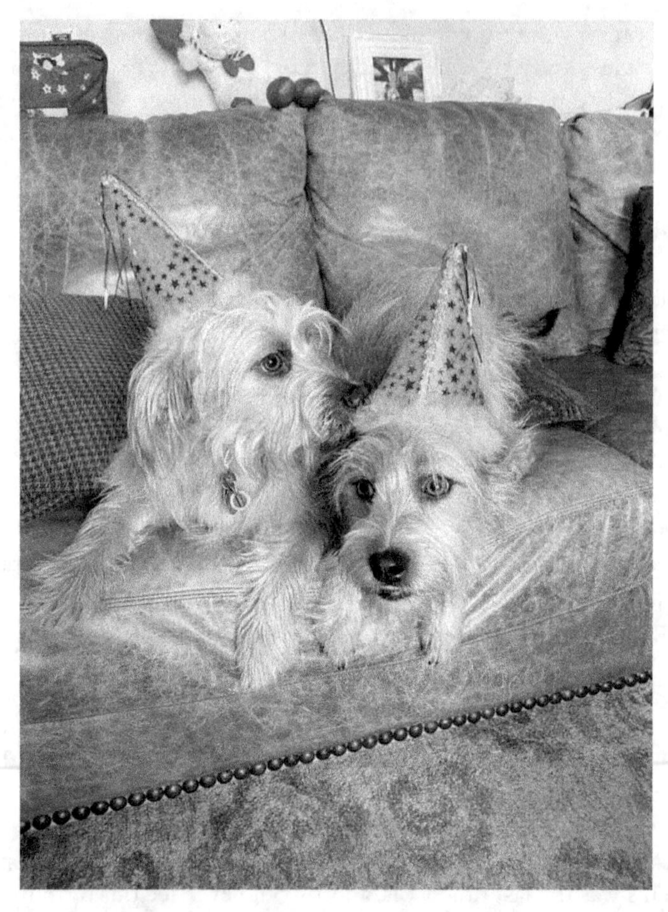

*"The dog was created specially for children.
He is the God of frolic."*

– Henry Ward

# CHAPTER 2
## *I KNEW – I WAS HOME*

After we left the foster house, I couldn't help but think about my mom and siblings. I wondered if I'd ever see them again. My dad? I never knew him, and I wasn't sure what had happened to him. My brother Colt and I sat quietly in the back seat of the car while the three ladies chatted away, discussing life, their plans, and their excitement about us. Meanwhile, I was filled with uncertainty. What would become of me? Yes, I was scared, but Colt reassured me that everything would be okay. Deep inside, I believed him, though the change was still overwhelming. You see, even though change is often good, the process can be frightening, especially when it happens so fast.

As we drove through the city, leaving behind the familiar sights and sounds of the foster home, I began to feel a sense of emptiness. Sure, I was destined to become a support dog, but at that moment, I needed support more than ever. I wasn't ready for this drastic shift, and I could only hope that these new humans would help me through it.

Eventually, the car stopped, and everyone hurried out. Colt and I were carefully lifted from the back seat and carried into a new home. It smelled different, looked different, and felt...new. An older man approached us with enthusiasm, particularly greeting my brother Colt as if he had won a lottery ticket. I waited for my turn, hoping for the same warm reception. After a moment, I was noticed and greeted, too, and then—suddenly—the man lay down on the floor, and Colt and I joined him, rolling around and playing. The ladies laughed, and for a brief moment, I felt a glimmer of peace.

But then it happened. I was picked up again, and I heard someone say, *"It's time to go home, Remi!"*

Wait... I thought I was home?

I looked at Colt, confusion filling my heart. I didn't understand. Weren't we a package deal? How could they separate us now? A knot formed in my stomach as I realized I would never see Colt again, just like I had been separated from my mother and siblings. Suddenly, everything felt heavy. I was going to have to face this new life alone.

The ladies said goodbye to the old man and woman, and we hopped back into the car, heading to a new destination. I sat in silence, feeling lost and scared. My life had changed in just a few hours, and I didn't know how to process it. Being a support dog, I would later learn, means understanding pain—and to help others, you must first feel it yourself.

When the car finally stopped again, I was carried through a garage and into yet another home. To my surprise, this one had other creatures—dogs like me, and two strange, smaller creatures I had never seen before. The humans set me down, allowing me to explore. It was a lot to take in, and I felt overwhelmed by all the newness. I sat there, staring at the unfamiliar faces, not sure if I was ready to engage.

The dogs, Gus and Tigger, seemed friendly. Gus was older, and I later learned he had some health challenges. He had trouble with his back and often made mistakes in the house. Tigger, on the other hand, was full of energy—feisty, playful, and always ready for an adventure. It didn't take long for Tigger and me to bond. Though the void left by my family still ached, it was comforting to have new friends to help me adjust.

Then there were the cats—those two peculiar creatures who liked to keep to themselves. They were quiet and sneaky, often hiding away from everyone. I learned quickly that they preferred solitude and didn't appreciate my attempts to play, but they were nice enough in their own way.

At first, I explored my new surroundings cautiously. There were so many smells to investigate, cozy corners to discover, and unfamiliar faces to observe. But as I settled in, I realized the most important part of this new chapter: my humans. It wasn't long before I sensed they needed me as much as I needed them. I could see it in their eyes, hear it in their voices. They were searching for something—something that I knew I could provide. Love. Joy. Peace.

I made it my mission, from that very first day, to remind them of the beauty of life. To show them how to live in the moment, to experience each day with joy, no matter how overwhelming the world could feel. My task was clear: I was here to help them, just as they were here to help me.

Days turned into weeks, and I began to see how much they needed me. Mom, as I started calling her, was always rushing, always moving, as if she had too many things to juggle. I would catch her staring off into the distance, her mind far away from where we were. When she looked like that, I'd nudge her leg, wag my tail, and remind her that I was there, right beside her. It always seemed to bring her back. She'd smile, bend down,

and give me a pat on the head, as if I was her little anchor in the sea of life.

Then there was Auntie Donna. She had a soft spot for me. Every time I walked into a room, she'd greet me with a cheerful, *"Hey there, handsome!"* Her gentle nature was a comfort in this new world, and I often found myself laying next to her as she chatted with Mom about their days.

Uncle Mike was different. He didn't say much, but he had a presence that made me feel safe. He had this routine where he would take Gus, Tigger, and me on short walks around the neighborhood. Each time we ventured out, I'd notice more about my surroundings—the birds chirping, the leaves rustling in the wind, the scent of freshly cut grass. I was slowly beginning to appreciate the beauty of my new life.

Tigger and Gus quickly became my companions in this new chapter of life. Tigger, the little firecracker, was always full of energy and opinions, darting ahead on walks like the whole world was his playground. He never stayed still, zigzagging from side to side, eager to explore every inch. Gus, in contrast, was more deliberate. He moved at a slower pace, carefully sniffing each corner and every tree, savoring the moment. I admired Gus's patience and calm demeanor, finding comfort in his steady presence, all while enjoying his dry sense of humor that always caught me by surprise.

But it wasn't just the dogs that helped me settle in—it was the quiet moments, too. The stillness of the night, when the house was calm, and I'd curl up at the foot of Mom's bed, listening to her breathing as she slept. It was in those moments that I realized I was no longer lost.

I wasn't scared anymore.

I had a family.

I had a home!

The cats, well, they remained a mystery. I'd watch them from a distance, their sleek bodies moving gracefully through the house. Every now and then, they'd glance my way, their eyes narrowing as if to say, *"Stay in your lane, dog."* I respected their space. They had their way of living, and I had mine.

The more time passed, the more I understood my place in this new world. My humans needed me, and I needed them. The emptiness I had felt when leaving my mother and siblings began to fade, replaced by the warmth of love and belonging. This was my home now, and I was exactly where I was meant to be.

One evening, as I lay by the fireplace, watching the flames flicker and dance, I realized how much my life had changed. The uncertainty and fear that had once gripped me had melted away. In its place was a deep sense of peace, a knowing that everything would be alright. I had a purpose here, with these humans, in this home.

And that's when I knew, I was home, *sigh*.

# CHAPTER 3
## *FINDING MY PLACE IN THE PACK*

The week flew by, and I was still trying to figure out who's who in this new family of mine. It's funny, but as much as I've been adopted into this home, I still haven't quite figured out who's in charge. There's Tigger, who *thinks* he's the Alpha, strutting around like he's the boss. But, in truth, I'm not convinced. In our home, there are two ladies and a man, along with three dogs (including me) and two strange creatures called cats that seem to have their own language. They call it *"Meow."* Have you heard of it? It's this bizarre, gibberish-sounding language that doesn't make much sense to me. All these cats do is lounge around and walk through the house meowing. I'm not sure who they're talking to or what they're trying to say, but they seem content in their mysterious, cat-like ways.

As for the humans, their language is starting to make sense to me, though I still don't always understand everything. You know what I mean? Some words are beginning to sound familiar, but the meanings are sometimes a bit blurry. For instance, I know "sit," but when they say "stay," I'm still figuring out how long that really means. Anyway, back to Tigger.

Tigger is a small dog, even smaller than me, and I'm already pretty small. I think he might be some kind of Terrier, but honestly, even he doesn't seem too sure. What's sad is that Tigger doesn't remember his mom, dad, or siblings, and I hope that never happens to me. Later on, I learned why—Tigger was rescued from a kill shelter after being found abandoned in the middle of a city in New Jersey. I guess that's why he's so cautious around people; you really have to earn his trust. It's understandable, given what he's been through.

I love my mom and siblings deeply, even though I've been adopted and live with this new family now. Family is family, and I hope I never forget where I came from. But despite his tough background, Tigger struts around like he owns the place. He's been here for a few years, and this is the only home he's ever known, so I guess he feels pretty comfortable acting like the leader.

Then there's Gus. Gus is old—really old—and smaller than both Tigger and me. Gus has his own agenda, and it mostly involves going outside every 15 minutes to pee. I'm not kidding, every 15 minutes! He's got this thing with his bladder because of his age. Did I mention Gus is old? Auntie Donna, one of the humans here, adopted Gus after his original human passed away a few years ago. He's a sweet old guy, quick with words, but sometimes he just seems lost. When Gus finishes doing his business outside, he doesn't come back in right away. Instead, he'll just sit there, rain or shine, staring off into the distance like he's thinking about something deep. It's as if he's lost in his own little world. I wonder if that's what happens when you get old—do you start to drift off into your thoughts? Poor Uncle Mike, the man of the house, often has to go outside and bring Gus back in, because Gus will just sit there forever if no one helps him.

As for the lady who adopted me, she says I should call her "Mom." It's strange because I already have a mom, and she lives far away. I'm not sure I'm ready to call this new lady "Mom" just yet, but she sure does take care of me like one. She makes sure I don't make a mess in the house, teaches me how to behave, takes me for walks, and gives me plenty of belly rubs. She even plays with me, gives me baths, and feeds me food that I'm still getting used to since I'm transitioning from puppy food to adult dog food. That's what moms do, right? They take care of you, love you, and make sure you feel safe.

One of my favorite things to do with this lady who wants me to call her Mom is going for walks around the neighborhood. For me, every step is an adventure. Every scent tells a story, and I love tugging on the leash to show her that there's something interesting ahead. It could be a patch of flowers, a squirrel darting up a tree, or even a new smell on the ground. I've noticed that she smiles when I get excited, and sometimes, I catch her looking at me with a little more joy in her eyes. I think I'm helping her see the world differently, a little more like I do—with wonder and excitement.

Sometimes, though, I see her staring at her phone or lost in thought, her face clouded with worry. That's when I nudge her with my nose or give a soft bark to bring her back to the present moment. It almost always works. She'll look down at me, laugh, and we'll continue walking. I like to think I'm helping her lighten the load, helping her realize that life is about being here, now, in this moment, and not getting lost in the worries of tomorrow.

At the end of each day, after our adventures around the neighborhood, my new Mom and I have a special routine. We curl up in bed together and watch television. She always rubs my belly, and we just enjoy the quiet time together. It reminds me of my birth mom and the way she always made sure I was taken care of. That sense of safety, of being cared for, it's something I try to give back. Being a support dog means understanding the importance of unconditional love, and how sometimes, all someone needs is to feel that someone is there for them, no matter what.

Tigger might think he's the Alpha of this household, but I'm beginning to see that love and care are what really keep a family strong. It's not about being in charge; it's about being there for each other. The man they call Uncle Mike, Auntie Donna, Gus, the mysterious meowing cats, and my new Mom—they're my family now. It's funny, even though this isn't where I started, it's starting to feel like home.

Not just in the physical sense, but in the way that truly counts. Home is where love surrounds you, where you can give love in return, and where joy is found in the simplest of moments. In this first week, I've learned so much, and it feels like my journey is only beginning. Life is good, and I'm ready for whatever adventures lie ahead.

As I lay here, drifting off to sleep, I know I'm exactly where I'm meant to be. This is my family now. I didn't know what to expect when I first arrived, but I've found love, comfort, and happiness in this new place. The unfamiliarity I once felt has faded, replaced by the warmth of a home where I belong.

And as I close my eyes, uncertain about who's really leading the pack, I realize it doesn't matter. Whether it's Tigger strutting around like he's the boss, or Gus moving through life at his own pace, none of it changes the way I feel. *Mom*—is making everything feel like home, just like my birth mom once did. Her gentle touch, her care, and her patience remind me every day that I'm safe and loved.

So, does it even matter who's in charge? Not at all. What matters is that I'm loved, and that's enough. Whether we're walking together, curled up on the couch, or just enjoying a quiet moment, the love in this home is what keeps me grounded. It's the anchor I didn't know I needed but have now found.

As I look up at the lady rubbing my tummy, a feeling of contentment washes over me. I don't have to worry about the past or what comes next. Right now, in this moment, everything is perfect. I give one last sigh, letting the calmness take over. Looking into her eyes, I feel the word I wasn't sure I was ready to say before rise naturally to the surface.

"Good night, Mommy," I whisper in my heart, and then I drift into a peaceful sleep, knowing I am truly home.

# CHAPTER 4
## *MONDAY'S*

We had just come back inside after our morning pee break. Tigger and I found our favorite spot on the couch while we waited for Uncle Mike to bring Gus in from the yard. Gus was outside again, lost in one of his deep, thoughtful moments. Auntie Donna had already left the house, but I knew she'd return later with treats for us, just like she always did. Meanwhile, Mom was downstairs getting ready for the day, and I could sense that something different was happening today. As Uncle Mike came inside with Gus, he joked, "Were you birdwatching out there?" Gus, as usual, just stared off into space, not bothered by much at all.

Mom came upstairs, and I could tell she was ready to go somewhere. I was a little confused. We had spent the whole week together, hanging out, and I had gotten used to the rhythm of our days. Then she sat down next to me on the couch, her hand resting gently on my head, and said, "I have a surprise for you."

Surprise? What does that even mean? Sometimes Mom talks to me like I understand everything she's saying, but honestly, I'm just a pup—I don't have a clue. Her words swirl around me like a breeze, and I try my best to catch their meaning, but I'm still learning. Before I could figure it out, Mom scooped me up and said, "We're going for a car ride."

Oh no, not another car ride! Again? I instantly felt a knot form in my stomach. Were we going to another new home? I had already been to three different homes in just one week, and the thought of another transition made me anxious. As Mom buckled me into my special seat in the car, my mind raced with worry. Would I have to leave behind Uncle Mike, Auntie Donna, and Tigger? What about Gus and the cats? I had just started to feel at home, and now, everything seemed uncertain again.

I sat in the car, completely consumed by all the "what ifs" running through my mind. Mom was talking to me, but I wasn't listening. I was too busy imagining the worst. What if I had done something wrong? Had I made a mess that I didn't know about? Did Uncle Mike or Auntie Donna get upset with me? I was spiraling, thinking about all the possible reasons why Mom might be taking me away.

Then, Mom said something that finally snapped me out of my thoughts. "Are you ready to see Colt?"

Wait, what? I needed to hear that again.

"We're going to see your brother Colt. Are you ready?"

I perked up and looked at her, my ears twitching as I processed what she said. We were going to see Colt? My brother? The one I thought I'd never see again after we were adopted? I couldn't believe it.

Mom repeated it again, this time with a smile in her voice, "Yes, we're going to see Colt, Grandma, and Paps."

Grandma and Paps? So, I have grandparents now too? For a moment, my heart raced with excitement. Maybe my birth mom would be there, and I could see her again. Maybe even my dad! Suddenly, all my worries melted away, replaced with anticipation and joy. I couldn't wait to see everyone.

As the car pulled into the driveway, I was so excited that I could barely sit still. The car door opened, and I jumped out, my paws hitting the ground with eagerness. An older lady—Colt's adoptive mom—came out to greet us, and the older man followed behind her. They were kind, but I ran right past them, scanning the area for my brother.

There he was! Colt! We greeted each other with wagging tails and playful nudges, but I couldn't stop searching for my birth family. Where were they? I looked at Colt with confusion, and he just tilted his head, wondering what I was doing. The older man, whom Colt called "Paps," suggested we go to the backyard to play. Colt and I raced to the yard, where we spent the afternoon chasing balls and rolling around in the grass.

But as much fun as I was having, I couldn't shake the feeling that something was missing. I had expected to see my birth mom and siblings, and it took me a while to understand that they weren't coming. Colt explained to me that he was the only one here from our litter, and that the old lady and old man were his adoptive parents. They were "Grandma" and "Paps" because my mom was their daughter. I hadn't realized that my new mom had adopted me into this family, connecting me to Colt in more ways than I had imagined.

At first, I felt a little sad. I had gotten myself so worked up in the car, expecting to see my whole family again, and now it wasn't happening. I had wasted so much time worrying and stressing about things that weren't real. Instead of enjoying the ride and Mom's company, I had let my fears take over.

That day, I learned an important lesson. As a support dog, my job is to help others stay present, but I had let myself get caught up in my own negative thoughts. It's something I still work on today. Worrying about the future or things that might not even happen doesn't bring peace—it only takes away from the joy of the present moment. I had spent that whole car ride imagining the worst when, in reality, something wonderful was waiting for me.

After we finished playing, I sat with Colt in the yard, reflecting on the day. Mondays had become my new favorite day because every Monday, I would get to see my brother and my adoptive grandparents. I had two homes now—both filled with love and joy.

Everything had worked out better than I could have imagined. I had been so focused on my fears that I hadn't seen the good that was unfolding right in front of me. Change can be scary, but it can also bring wonderful surprises if you're patient and open to them.

As I curled up with Mom that night, tired but happy, I realized something important: Life is full of surprises, and sometimes the best thing you can do is stop worrying, live in the moment, and trust that everything will be okay. In fact, I need to start thinking that anything and everything that happens to me is good, and by accepting the world as it is, not only will I benefit, but those around me will feel the positive change too. My calm acceptance can be a source of peace, not just for myself, but for everyone I love.

I looked up at Mom, who was gently rubbing my tummy, her eyes soft and full of love, and whispered in my heart, "I'm home."

In that moment, I knew that no matter where I went, no matter what happened, as long as I kept this sense of peace and love, everything would be just fine. Because home isn't just a place—it's the feeling of being loved and giving love in return. It's knowing that every experience, every change, is a part of life's journey, and as long as we face it with an open heart, we will always find our way.

# CHAPTER 5
## *THE MEXICAN STANDOFF*

Have you ever heard of a Mexican standoff? Uncle Mike was telling us a story about one—how Colt and Tigger first met—and he described it just like the iconic standoff scene from *The Good, the Bad, and the Ugly* movie. You know, the one where the hero, villain, and wildcard face off in a tense three-way duel, each one waiting for the other to make the first move. Uncle Mike was really into it, saying that Tigger was the hero in this story, standing tall, ready to defend his territory.

His version was entertaining, no doubt, but I remember the event quite differently.

It happened just a few days ago, after Mom and I had visited Colt, Grandma, and Papa at their home. This time, they were coming over to visit us, and Mom wanted to introduce Colt to Tigger, Gus, and the two mysterious creatures known as cats—who speak a language I'm still trying to figure out. "Meow!" I think I'm getting closer to pronouncing it correctly, but honestly, I still have no idea what it means.

Anyway, back to the story. Grandma came into the house first, and naturally, Tigger, Gus, and I ran up to greet her. In our doggy language, licking someone's face is a way of giving affection, so we all showered her with kisses. There's so much,

I'm still learning, and it feels like I have so much knowledge to share.

*"Squirrel!"*

Just kidding! No distractions. I'm typing away on Dad's computer, and Dad is another story for another time. It's still too soon to talk about him. Now, where was I?

Oh yes, Grandma came in, and after we gave her kisses, Papa followed, and we all ran up to him for more affectionate greetings. Then came Colt. I was so excited to see my brother! I barked happily as he entered the house, but Gus just sat there looking between me and Colt, tilting his head back and forth in confusion. It was like he couldn't quite figure out what was going on. Why were there two of me?

Now, we've already talked about Tigger being the self-appointed boss of the house. He wasn't about to let another dog stroll in and dominate his territory, especially not one as tough as Colt. You see, Colt's got a reputation for being a strong-willed and fearless dog. Growing up, I remember Colt and one of our other brothers getting into some serious fights. My birth mom always had to step in to break them up. Colt came out of those squabbles even tougher than before. He's older than the rest of us, and I'm the baby of the litter, so I always learned to avoid conflict. But Colt? He fought his way through life, which probably explains his fearless attitude.

When Tigger saw Colt, things took a turn. Tigger immediately bared his teeth and let out a low, mean growl. Colt, on the other hand, just sat there grinning at Tigger. It wasn't that Colt was being cocky; it's just that Tigger is smaller than him, and Colt doesn't take anyone's rudeness lightly. The tension was thick. Tigger, growling and showing his teeth, and Colt, smiling like he had all the time in the world—neither one of them was willing to make the first move. It was the perfect standoff.

Gus and I sat there watching, unsure of what was going to happen next. Gus, who usually preferred to stay out of drama, looked more interested than I'd ever seen him. In fact, I think this was the most excitement Gus had seen in a long time.

Suddenly, out of the corner of my eye, I saw Papa stepping toward Tigger, probably thinking he could scoop him up and diffuse the situation. But Tigger wasn't having it. He snapped at Papa, and we all frozen. Papa, surprised, calmly said, "Tigger, that wasn't nice. Leave him alone."

I couldn't believe it! Tigger, the tough little dog who thought he ruled the house, had just snapped at Papa. Even Gus was wide-eyed, his usual laid-back expression momentarily replaced with interest.

Realizing that things were escalating fast, Tigger huffed and made his way toward the door, wanting to go outside to cool off. We all followed him, which was good because the tension in the house needed to be diffused quickly.

Out in the yard, Tigger sat by himself for a moment, still visibly upset. I went over to check on him, and that's when he told me why he'd been so angry. He explained that Colt looked a lot like me, and he was confused. Tigger had never seen two dogs that looked so similar, and it made him feel threatened. Plus, Tigger rarely left the house, only going out for short walks around the neighborhood, so he hadn't met many new dogs before. The unfamiliarity of Colt's appearance had thrown him off and snapping at Papa had been an impulse born out of frustration and confusion.

As the afternoon wore on, we all played together outside, and the tension between Colt and Tigger gradually eased. Despite his tough demeanor, Colt wasn't looking for a fight, and Tigger quickly realized Colt wasn't here to take over his territory. By the end of the day, they were running around the yard like old friends, as if their earlier standoff had never happened.

Uncle Mike's story was entertaining, but the real takeaway wasn't about some grand Wild West showdown. It was about how misunderstandings can easily spiral out of control if we let them. We often jump to conclusions, seeing others as threats or feeling the need to defend our space. But more often than not, we simply need to step back, give things time, and let situations cool off on their own.

Now, Colt and Tigger are the best of friends, and we all live together peacefully. Even Paps wasn't upset with Tigger, and they quickly returned to their usual bond. While Uncle Mike still calls that day the "Mexican standoff" of our household, I see it differently. It was a moment of growth for all of us. We learned that things aren't always as they seem, and sometimes all it takes is a little patience and the willingness to give others—and ourselves—a chance to see things from a different perspective.

For me, the best part was seeing everyone come together. It meant Colt could visit more often, and I could go to his house too. What a relief to know that despite their rocky start, Colt and Tigger found common ground. They both realized there was no reason to fight—there was enough love and space for everyone.

That day taught me an important lesson: most conflicts arise from misunderstandings. But if we take a moment to cool off, talk things through, and try to understand the other side, we can often find peaceful resolutions. Tigger initially felt threatened, but once he realized Colt wasn't a rival, he let his guard down and relaxed.

Now, the tension between Colt and Tigger is a distant memory. The four of us—me, Colt, Tigger, and Gus—have become a happy little pack. We play, nap, and live together in harmony. Each of us has our quirks, but we're united by the love we share in our family. With all of us here, the house feels complete, and there's no room left for misunderstandings.

As for Uncle Mike's "Mexican standoff"? It turned out to be nothing more than a brief moment of confusion, the kind of misunderstanding that could have easily escalated. In the end, there were no heroes or villains—just a group of dogs learning how to coexist. And we're all better for it.

*Oh, I've got to go—Dad's calling me! Stay* "MEOW"! Whatever that means...

# CHAPTER 6
## *BIRDWATCH*

As a support dog, I'm still learning to understand when someone is in need of comfort. Sometimes, it's obvious—a sad look, a heavy sigh, or tears. But other times, when someone is hurting, they do their best to hide it, keeping their pain inside. That's when I have to rely on my instincts to sense when something is wrong, and offer comfort in whatever way I can. One of my greatest teachers in this was Gus. I like to think I was Gus's first support dog.

Now, Gus is old—really old. Some would say he's near the end of his journey. But if I've learned anything from Gus, it's that age is just a number, and we all have something to teach and share, no matter how long we've been around. Gus has his quirks, like anyone else. He's a bit slow, and sometimes he just stares off into the distance like he's lost in another world. Tigger doesn't get it—he mostly ignores Gus, thinking he's strange. But I wondered, was Gus really strange, or was there something about him that Tigger just didn't take the time to understand?

I decided that I was going to try to understand Gus. I wanted to know why he sat in the middle of the yard, staring off into space like he was deep in thought. What was going through his mind?

One day, we were outside in the backyard. Tigger and I were chasing each other, having fun, while Gus did his usual thing—sitting in the grass, looking lost in thought. Uncle Mike called us to come inside because it was starting to rain. Tigger immediately trotted off, and I was about to follow, but I stopped and looked back at Gus.

He was just sitting there, still as a stone, staring up at the sky as the rain started to fall. Drops hit his face, but he didn't move. He looked like he was... at peace, as if the rain was something he had been waiting for. I tried to bark and get his attention, "Whoof, whoof!" But Gus didn't respond. He just kept sitting there, soaking in the moment.

So, instead of going inside, I turned back around and sat beside him. I looked up at the sky, trying to see what he was seeing. But all I saw were clouds and raindrops. I didn't quite understand why Gus found so much peace in that moment, but I stayed with him anyway. We sat there together, just the two of us, until Uncle Mike came out, shaking his head with a smile.

"Remi, what are you doing? Bird-watching with Gus?"

Uncle Mike picked us both up and carried us inside. Tigger was already on the couch, looking at me like I was crazy for sitting out in the rain. After Uncle Mike dried us off, I curled up next to Tigger, warm and cozy, while Gus found a spot next to Auntie Donna. She petted him gently as he stared blankly at the TV. Yet, Gus looked content.

I didn't stop thinking about that rainy day. I wanted to understand what Gus saw when he sat in the yard, staring off into the distance. Every time we went outside after that, Gus would do the same thing—sit there quietly, not moving, while the rest of us played. And every time, I would sit beside him, watching, waiting, trying to understand.

Weeks went by like this, and every time Auntie Donna, Uncle Mike, or Mom would come to call us inside, I'd follow Gus's lead. As I sat beside him, I started to notice things I hadn't before—the beauty of the trees swaying in the wind, the different songs the birds sang, the way the clouds moved across the sky. The world was always changing, always moving, but in a slow, gentle way that I'd never paid attention to before. Gus seemed to understand that, and I was learning too.

One day, as we sat together in the yard, I noticed a cloud in the sky that looked just like a big dog bone. I couldn't help but say, "Gus, do you see that cloud? It looks like a bone!" To my surprise, Gus responded, quietly but clearly, "Yup."

That was the first time Gus had ever said anything to me. And from that moment on, we started talking more, though our conversations were simple and slow. Gus didn't say much, but what he did say mattered.

Over time, I realized that Gus wasn't lost in thought at all. He was deeply connected to the world around him. He wasn't sitting there thinking about the past or worrying about the future—he was living in the moment, appreciating the simple beauty of life. The rain, the trees, the birds, the sky—they were all part of the present, and Gus was fully immersed in it.

Gus taught me something incredibly valuable: being still is not the same as being lost. Sometimes, the most peaceful moments come from simply sitting still and appreciating the world as it is. While I had always been excited by running around and playing, I learned from Gus that there's a whole world to discover when you stop and look around.

Now, whenever we go outside, I always make time to sit with Gus. We don't always talk, but we sit together, watching the clouds and feeling the breeze. It's become our little ritual, and it reminds me that life doesn't always have to be full of action to be meaningful. Sometimes, the most profound moments come when you're just sitting still, enjoying the world.

As a support dog, I've realized that part of my job is to help others see what Gus has taught me—that even in the quietest moments, there is beauty and peace. And sometimes, the best way to support someone is simply to be there with them, sitting in silence, reminding them that they're not alone.

Gus may be old, but he's wise. And I'm grateful for everything he's taught me about life, about being present, and about finding peace in the simplest of moments. I like to think I was Gus's first support dog, but the truth is, he's been a teacher to me in more ways than I can count.

Now, every time we sit together, I look at the world through Gus's eyes, and I understand: everything is okay. Life is beautiful, just as it is.

So, it's okay to "Birdwatch." Oh, I've got to run... Mom and I are heading out

for a walk.

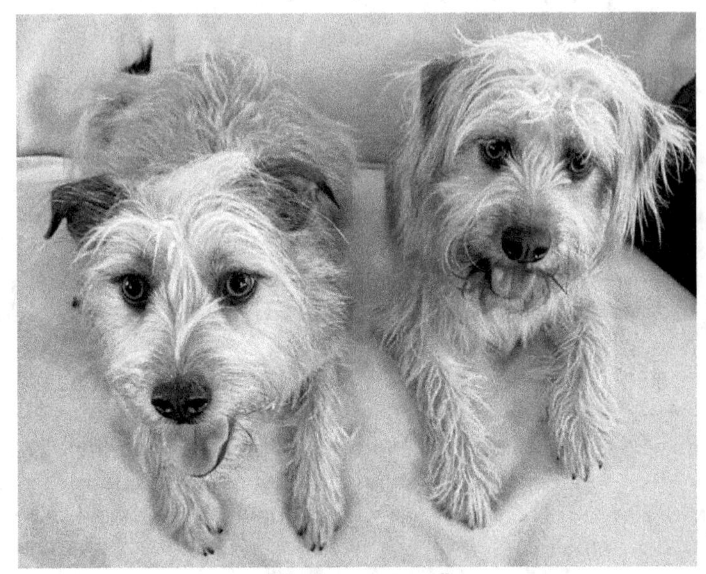



*"No one appreciates the very special genius of your
conversation as the dog does."*

– Christopher Morley

# CHAPTER 7
## *SUNSETS & RAINBOWS*

As I grow older, I'm starting to understand more about humans and their emotions. Life isn't always sunny for them, just like it isn't for me. Some days are rainy, and not just because of the weather. We all have our ups and downs, and as a support dog, I've come to learn that I'm here for a reason—maybe many reasons. Some dogs like me are here to provide companionship, unconditional love, and to reduce loneliness. We help boost the mental well-being of our humans, offering them a sense of connection. It's more than just wagging tails and belly rubs—it's about being there when they need us the most.

Support dogs like me can help manage anxiety and chronic stress by just being present. Spending time with us releases the chemicals that make humans feel happy—serotonin, dopamine, and oxytocin—while reducing stress. We can even help those with post-traumatic stress disorder (PTSD), waking them from nightmares or comforting them during panic attacks. And for those with bipolar disorder, we offer grounding and emotional balance, helping them regain focus when life feels overwhelming.

We're more than just animals on leashes—we're partners in this journey of life. It took me a while to understand my role fully, but one day, I realized why I was needed in Mom's life.

Mom had been through a lot. She had bad relationships in the past and was never able to find the right person. She didn't have children because of those experiences, and that's when I came into her life. She didn't adopt me just to have a dog around the house—she adopted me because she needed someone to love and care for. Someone to be there for her. And that's when I knew why I was home with Mom. My purpose was clear: I was here to help her through the tough times, to bring joy to her life, and to remind her that love is always near, even when things feel hard.

I'd overhear conversations between Auntie Donna and Mom. Mom would talk about how some of the men she had dated were controlling and, at times, abusive. It hurt to hear, and I wished I could've been there to protect her from those bad moments. I know I would've stood by her side, and maybe even taken a bite out of the bad ones! But those times have passed, and Mom has grown stronger because of them. She learned a lot about herself through those tough experiences, and now, her heart is full of love and joy. I like to believe I played a small part in helping her realize that life can get better.

Since I've come into her life, Mom has had someone to love unconditionally, and that's me. I'm here for her, no matter what, and she knows it. Our bond has helped her overcome the tough nights, the loneliness, and the anxiety. Now, she has someone to look forward to at the end of the day, and so do I. We curl up in bed together and watch our favorite episodes of The King of Queens, falling asleep to the sound of laughter. Every night, I'm reminded that I'm exactly where I'm meant to be.

Mom and I go everywhere together—well, almost everywhere. I can't go to her workplace, but I've been on plenty of car rides to the beach, restaurants, hotels, and soon, we're even going on a plane ride to New Mexico to visit Dad's friend, Craig. Oh, and about Dad—well, that's a story for another time. But trust me, I'll tell you all about him soon.

As I've learned more about life and people, I've come to see myself as more than just a dog. I'm a little boy in my mom's arms, and that's a role I take seriously.

The other day, I heard Mom talking to Auntie Donna. She said, "This morning, I stood in the kitchen and watched Remi as I gave him his morning treat. I remember when he was so small that he had to climb the stairs, one paw at a time. I used to cut up his treats because they were too big for him to chew. Now, he's so much bigger, and those stairs seem small under his paws. I just wonder if he knows how much I love him."

Without missing a beat, Auntie Donna turned to me and then looked back at Mom. "You know Remi loves you. Just look at him—he follows you around like he's your lost kid!" Auntie Donna was right. I love Mom more than anything, and I'll always be there to remind her of that.

Even on those rainy days, I'm here for Mom, wagging my tail and ready to bring a little sunshine back into her life. When she's feeling down, I remind her that after the rain, there's always a rainbow. And if she's lucky, maybe she'll even spot a squirrel!

Being here for Mom isn't about fixing her problems—it's about being present, offering her love, and showing her that she's never alone. It's a lesson I hope everyone can carry with them, long after the rain has passed.

Because in the end, there's always sunshine behind the clouds. The rain is only temporary, a moment to help us reflect on what's possible. And when the rain disappears, the sun will come out, and a rainbow will appear, reminding us that everything is going to be okay.

Life isn't perfect, but there's always hope. And when the clouds' part and the rainbow shines through, we realize that love and joy are always just around the corner. All we have to do is wait for the storm to pass.

It's raining, so I'm signing off for now. I'm going to curl up with Mom in bed and watch The King of Queens. Oh, and don't forget—always chase after sunsets and rainbows, not rainstorms.

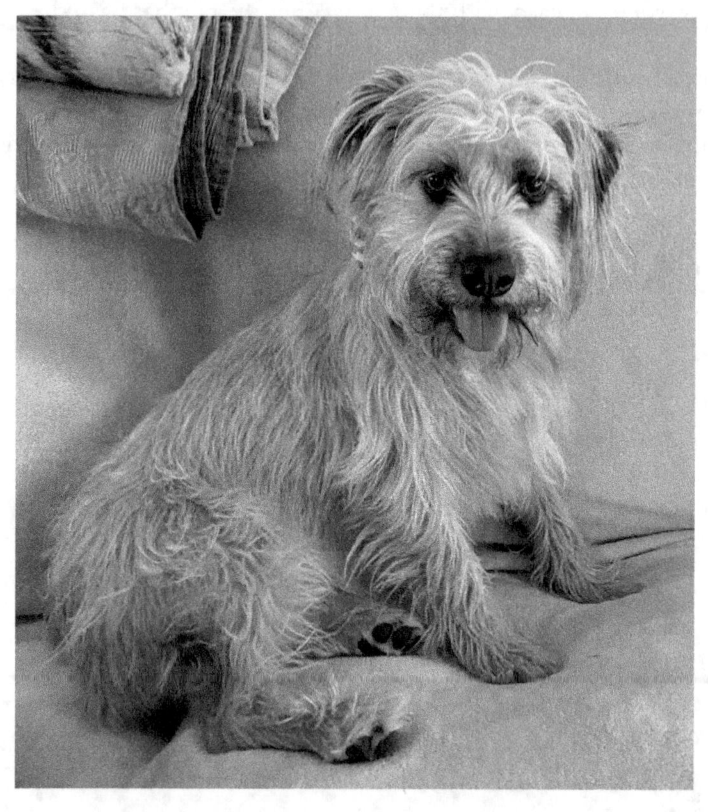

"The dog has got more fun out of man than man
has got out of the dog, for man is the more
laughable of the two animals."

– James Thurber

# CHAPTER 8
## *HOLIDAYS*

In the beginning, I wasn't a big fan of Thanksgiving and Christmas. For a lot of people, holidays are filled with joy and celebration, but for those of us who are adoptees, or have experienced foster care, they can feel isolating. Growing up as an adoptee in a big, loving family, I felt like an imposter. While everyone around me enjoyed the warmth and togetherness, I felt disconnected, like I didn't truly belong.

It wasn't that my adoptive family didn't love me—they did, deeply. But I couldn't shake the feeling that I was there to fill a void, to help make their lives feel complete. Everyone expected me to feel nothing but "grateful" for being "saved" from the foster care system, for having a home, and for all the gifts under the Christmas tree. But no one ever asked about my life before I was adopted, about the pieces of my past that stayed with me, like shadows I couldn't ignore. They didn't understand that my story didn't start the day they brought me home.

As the holidays rolled around each year, I found myself questioning more and more why Mom always felt the need to dress me up for special occasions. "Seriously, why are these things on me?" I'd think, as she'd put silly hats and costumes on me for every holiday. It started with my first Fourth of July—Mom decided I needed a funny hat to celebrate. Then came Halloween, when she dressed me up as some kind of scary monster. But, come on—how scary can I be? I'm adorable, and nothing can change that.

Christmas was the worst. Every year, Mom and Auntie Donna would collaborate on how the entire family should dress. And yes, I mean the entire family—Tigger, Gus, Uncle Mike, Auntie Donna, Mom, and me—all dressed up in matching outfits like we were part of some kind of circus act. And the cats? They never had to wear a thing! Tigger told me it was because they were special, but I didn't get it.

I always did my best to smile for Mom, though. One year, even Grandma, Papa, and Colt joined in, and Mom got them matching outfits too. We all took pictures, and after it was over, the family gathered to open presents and reminisce about past holidays. As I sat there, surrounded by my new family, my thoughts drifted to my birth mom. What if she was here to share these moments with me? Maybe that's why the holidays felt so difficult. Even though I was happy with my new family, a part of me always felt missing.

I wasn't able to fully enjoy the holidays, even though I tried. There was always this lingering sense of loss, a piece of my past that wasn't there to share in the joy. Yes, I had Colt in my life, and we got to see each other, but deep down, I resented my adoptive relatives for something they couldn't control— their privilege. They had the privilege of sitting around the table, talking about who looked like who, sharing stories of their roots, their names, their memories. They had a shared history, while I was the one they "chose" to join the family.

"When we got Remi..."

"We chose you, like our own..."

Those words, meant to be comforting, sometimes felt like salt in a wound. It was as if they believed my life started the day I was adopted, as if everything that happened before didn't matter. During holiday gatherings, I'd hear whispers and laughter, and I couldn't help but wonder if they were talking about me. Maybe they thought, "His real mom didn't want him," or "He's lucky to be here." Those thoughts haunted me, making me feel like an outsider even as I sat in the middle of a loving family.

I acknowledged my losses, but I also counted my blessings. Even though I wasn't always able to be present, I knew I had gained a lot in my new life. But there was always that piece of me that felt out of place, like I didn't belong at someone else's holiday table.

For adoptees and those who've been through foster care, grieving that loss is a lifelong process. It's okay to take that journey at our own pace, and to define when and where we feel ready to celebrate. Holidays are still hard for me, but they're getting easier. My adoptive family has been there for me every step of the way, and as I grow, I'm learning to embrace the moments, even when they're difficult.

One of the hardest lessons I've had to learn as a support dog is that I'm not perfect—and that's okay. None of us are. We all have a past, filled with both good and bad moments, and part of my job is to help my family navigate theirs. The more I learn about myself and my role in this family, the more I realize that it's okay to miss the people and pieces of my past. They're still with me, in my memories, and they always will be.

So, when I find myself dressed up like a clown for another holiday photo, I remind myself that it's not about the silly outfit or the perfect picture. It's about the love that surrounds me, the connections I've made, and the joy I bring to my family—even on the hard days.

Today, I'm getting ready for another family picture. Yes, I'm in my clownish Christmas outfit again, and yes, I'm smiling. Not because I love the outfit, but because I'm finally learning to accept and embrace the life I have now, quirks and all.

Before I go, let me leave you with this: Life isn't perfect, and neither are we. It's okay to miss the people and places we've lost, but don't let that stop you from embracing the moments you have now. Don't be a clown about it—make the most of what you have, and remember that love, even when it feels complicated, is always worth celebrating.

Alright, I've got to run. The family picture is about to happen, and I'm ready to style and profile in my Christmas outfit!

Woooo!

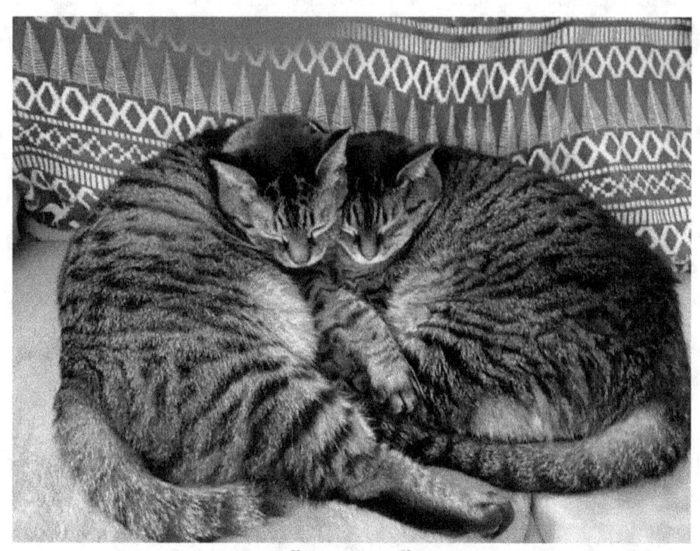



"*Animals have come to mean so much in our lives. We live in a fragmented and disconnected culture. Politics are ugly, religion is struggling, technology is stressful, and the economy is unfortunate. What's one thing that we have in our lives that we can depend on? A dog or a cat loving us unconditionally, every day, very faithfully.*"

– Jon Katz

# CHAPTER 9
## *THE RAT PACK*

Winter is fun, but you know what's even better? Spring and summer. Why? Because I get to play outside more with Tigger and Gus. We've even started calling ourselves "The Rat Pack." Gus, Tigger, and I spend hours outside when the weather is warm, and let me tell you, Gus is always scheming something. In fact, all winter long, Gus had been planning a big escape from the backyard, something we called "The Great Escape."

It all started last year when Gus figured out the weak spots around the fence. Gus is older and wiser, so he spent a lot of time observing everything, while Tigger and I were more focused on playing and chasing each other around. Gus noticed that the dirt on the southern side of the yard, by the fence, was softer and easier to dig through. He started digging there last summer but had to stop when the frost came. He told us he was preparing for when the ground thawed—come spring, we'd make our big break.

Gus's plan wasn't just about escaping for the fun of it. No, he had a mission. He wanted to get to the local park, a place he believed offered a perfect view of the stars. "The stars," he said, "look so much better when you're out in the open, with no lights from the house to block them." Gus was determined, and with each cold day that passed in winter, we waited eagerly for spring.

By the time spring finally rolled around, Gus had his plan in full swing. His blueprint for escape was a masterclass in strategy, or at least that's what he told us. He'd named the tunnels he planned to dig after the tunnels from a movie he once heard Uncle Mike talk about—The Great Escape. The three tunnels were called Tom, Dick, and Harry. Gus said they were essential to our plan: "Tom" was the decoy, the tunnel most likely to be discovered by Uncle Mike. "Dick" and "Harry," however, were our real tickets out. They were going to be dug under the tree line on the south side of the yard, where Uncle Mike wouldn't be able to see us working.

Gus had it all worked out. He would dig "Dick," Tigger would be responsible for "Harry," and I, being the youngest and most innocent-looking, was given the task of digging "Tom." My role was crucial because if Uncle Mike caught me digging, he'd just chalk it up to youthful curiosity. Meanwhile, Gus and Tigger would be busy digging the real escape routes. The plan was solid, and we estimated it would take about an hour to complete the tunnels if we worked together. Someone would always have to keep an eye out for Uncle Mike, though—he was known for patrolling the backyard.

The day of the escape finally arrived. We were all ready. It was 7:00 a.m., and the air was crisp. Mom and Auntie Donna were still asleep, and Uncle Mike was busy with his morning coffee, oblivious to our scheming. The door opened, and we darted outside, each of us heading to our assigned tunnels. I ran over to "Tom," the tunnel Gus had started before the frost came, and immediately began digging. My heart raced as the dirt flew behind me. I wondered what would happen if we got caught, but there was no turning back now.

I could hear Gus and Tigger working on their tunnels, and before I knew it, Tigger called out, "We're through!" I stopped digging and ran over to the tree line, where Gus and Tigger were both emerging from the other side of the fence. They had successfully dug through, and now it was my turn to follow them.

We were free!

The first part of the mission was complete, and we sprinted toward the park, weaving between houses to avoid being seen. Gus was leading the way, determined to reach his perfect stargazing spot. Tigger and I followed, trying to stay as quiet as possible. Along the way, I couldn't help but notice people looking at us—three dogs running freely through the neighborhood without any humans in sight. Gus told us to focus on the goal and not get distracted, but my stomach rumbled. We hadn't gotten our morning treats, and I was starting to feel the hunger, but I didn't dare complain. I didn't want Gus and Tigger to think I was weak.

When we finally reached the park, it was still early, and there were some kids playing on the swings. We took cover under the trees, waiting for nightfall. Gus had told us that once the sun went down, we'd have the whole park to ourselves, and he could show us the stars like we'd never seen them before.

But there was one problem—I was really hungry. I didn't want to break the silence, but the lack of treats was starting to bother me. We lay there, hidden under the trees, watching the kids play. Time seemed to stretch on forever. Then, suddenly, I heard something that made my ears perk up.

A familiar voice.

I turned to look and saw her—Mom. She was calling my name! My heart leaped with excitement. Without thinking, I bolted from our hiding spot, forgetting all about the mission. Gus and Tigger tried to call me back, but I was already running full speed toward Mom. I missed her so much, and I figured if she was here, she might have treats!

As I reached her, Mom knelt down and hugged me. Her voice was soft but a little worried. "There you are, Remi. We've been looking everywhere for you."

Auntie Donna and Uncle Mike appeared a few moments later, their eyes scanning the park. They quickly spotted where Gus and Tigger were hiding, and Uncle Mike called them over. There was no point in hiding anymore. The mission was over.

That night, after we returned home, we all sat together in the living room. Uncle Mike gave each of us a treat, and Mom laughed as she retold the story of how she found me running toward her like I hadn't seen her in years. I curled up next to her, content.

Gus's "Great Escape" hadn't gone as planned, but I learned something important that day: sometimes, no matter how big the adventure, nothing beats the feeling of being home. Sure, we missed seeing the stars that night, but I realized that I didn't need to escape the backyard to feel free. Being with Mom, Tigger, Gus, Auntie Donna, Uncle Mike and yes the cats—that's where I truly belong.

And you know what? Gus didn't even seem upset that the plan fell apart. As we all curled up together that night, I looked over at him, and he gave me a knowing smile. "We'll get another chance," he said. "But for now, let's just enjoy being together."

And I couldn't agree more.

The Rat Pack may have been foiled in their Great Escape, but at the end of the day, we realized that sometimes the greatest adventure is simply being with the ones you love.

Alright, I'm signing off now because we're about to watch The Great Escape! See you later!

And I couldn't agree more.

**The Rat Pack may have been foiled in their Great Escape, but at the end of the day, we realized that sometimes the greatest adventure is simply being with the ones you love.**

Alright, I'm signing off now because we're about to watch *The Great Escape!*

# CHAPTER 10
## *ONE STEP*

It all started one summer day when Mom decided we should try hiking. I could sense her hesitation from the start. As she talked to Auntie Donna, I overheard her expressing doubts. "What if it's too hard for him?" she asked, her voice tinged with uncertainty. But I wasn't worried, not even a little. After all, I'm a support dog—hiking? Climbing a trail? I knew we could handle it. More importantly, I knew she could handle it. So, with a wag of my tail and a determined spring in my step, I took the lead, ready to show Mom that we could conquer anything, one step at a time.

The trail wound through the woods, with tall trees towering above us, and the fresh scent of earth and pine filling the air. I took the lead, eagerly sniffing out the best path, my tail wagging with each new discovery. The sun peeked through the branches, creating dappled patterns on the ground, and the wind carried hints of damp moss, making my nose twitch with excitement. As the trail steepened, I glanced back at Mom, giving her a look of encouragement, as if to say, "Come on, we've got this."

The hike wasn't easy. There were moments when the path was so steep that I had to slow down and focus on each step, carefully finding my footing. Mom, too, struggled at times. I saw her pause, catching her breath, eyes scanning the endless incline before us. But each time she stopped, I waited for her, wagging my tail and nudging her leg to remind her that we were in this together. I've learned that my role as a support

dog isn't just about offering comfort—sometimes, it's about pushing forward when things get tough and showing my mom that she can keep going, one step at a time.

Not every day is about climbing mountains, though. Some days are for resting, for lying in soft grass and watching clouds drift by. I've taught my mom that it's okay to take breaks, to breathe deeply, and just be. On those quiet days, we sit together in the backyard or the park, listening to the world around us.

Mom talks about her day, her worries, and her dreams. I may not understand every word, but I'm there, leaning against her to show that I'm always listening.

Mom often tells me how much I help her, how I bring her comfort and joy. But the truth is, she helps me too. She's shown me kindness, patience, and care. In return, I've tried to teach her how to slow down, to savor life's simple pleasures. Whether it's enjoying a belly rub, a tasty treat, or simply lying in the grass watching the world go by, I've learned that sometimes, the best thing you can do is pause and take it all in.

As we climbed that trail together, I realized something important: everyone has their own journey, their own path. Life isn't a race. Some people might seem ahead, while others might appear to be behind. But I've learned that it doesn't matter how fast you're moving, as long as you're moving forward, one step at a time.

I could see that realization dawning in Mom's eyes too. The hesitation and uncertainty that she carried at the beginning of the hike were slowly fading. With each step, she found her own rhythm, her own pace. It wasn't about reaching the top as fast as possible—it was about embracing the journey, taking things one step at a time.

There were tough moments, though. Times when Mom's legs trembled, and I could see the weariness on her face. She looked like she wanted to give up, the steep incline seemingly too much to handle. But I kept pushing forward, keeping my nose to the ground, paws steady as I dug into the dirt. I knew that if I didn't give up, neither would she. And sure enough, with every step, her confidence grew. I could see the change in her—she found strength, joy, and a peace that hadn't been there before.

By the time we reached the top, the sun was setting, casting a golden light across the landscape. We stood there in silence, soaking in the moment. Mom's breathing was steady now, and her face was calm. I sat beside her, wagging my tail slowly, feeling the cool breeze on my fur. We didn't need to say anything— this moment was everything.

It was in that quiet moment that I understood something essential: life isn't about racing to the finish line or comparing your progress to others. It's about taking things one step at a time, appreciating the journey, and finding joy in the little things. Mom had been hesitant, unsure if she could handle the hike. But in the end, it wasn't about being the fastest or the strongest—it was about showing up, trying, and believing in herself. As her support dog, I couldn't have been prouder.

Since that day, we've gone on more hikes together. Each time, we find new trails, new challenges, and new moments of peace. Some days, the path is easy, and we chat as we walk, enjoying the time together. Other days, the trail is hard, and we have to dig deep to keep going. But no matter what, we take it one step at a time.

On the days when we don't hike, we rest. Sometimes we lie in the grass, watching the clouds and pointing out funny shapes. Other times, we sit quietly in the backyard, listening to the birds and feeling the warmth of the sun. These moments remind us that it's okay to take a break, to slow down, and simply breathe.

I've learned that life is all about balance—pushing forward when you need to, but knowing when to rest, too. It's about being there for the people you love, even when the journey is tough. And most importantly, it's about believing in yourself, trusting that no matter where you are, you're exactly where you're meant to be.

So, if you ever feel like life's trail is too steep, remember: one step at a time is all it takes. You don't need to rush to the top, and you don't need to compare yourself to anyone else. Just keep going, enjoy the view along the way, and when you need to, pause, breathe, and rest.

Because whether you're climbing mountains or lying in the grass, there's always beauty in the journey. And in the end, it's not about how fast you get there—it's about the memories you make, the lessons you learn, and the love you share along the way.

One step at a time—that's all it takes.

Alright, friends, it's time for me to sign off. After a long day of adventure and a story well told, I'm off to curl up next to Mom, maybe sneak in a few extra belly rubs while we relax. Remember, no matter how steep the trail, just take it one step at a time. Until next time, keep wagging and enjoying the journey!

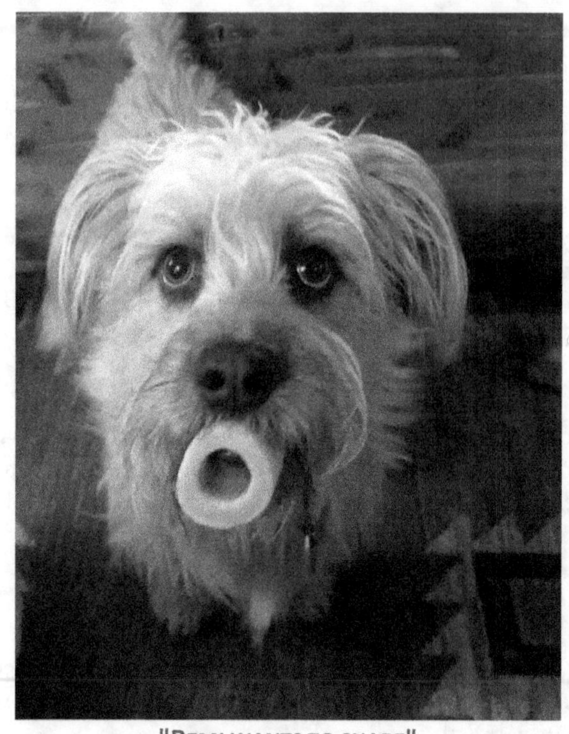

"REMI WANTS TO SHARE"

*"They [dogs] never talk about themselves but listen to you while you talk about yourself and keep up an appearance of being interested in the conversation."*

— Jerome K. Jerome

# CHAPTER 11
## *DUDE*

Life is good. Every day with Mom is an adventure, a journey we walk together. We've explored trails, chased sunsets, and discovered so many beautiful things about the world and ourselves. We've learned that life isn't a race but a path that we walk, one step at a time.

On Mondays, I get to visit my brother Colt, Grandma, and Papa. We play in the backyard, chasing each other, and sometimes Papa gets down on the floor to wrestle with us. I even get to sleep over sometimes, which means extra time with Colt and his family. In between, I have Gus, Tigger, Uncle Mike, Auntie Donna, and of course, the two cats. "Meow!"—I still don't know what that means, but I'll figure it out one day. Life is good, right?

Wrong.

Mom decided to start dating again. Why? Life was perfect just the way it was—Mom and me, plus everyone else. But dating? That was something I didn't understand. As a support dog, my job is to give unconditional love and push Mom in the right direction, like when we go hiking and she gets tired— I'm her spirit, the one who helps her keep going. But now, I was feeling selfish. Instead of spending nights curled up with Mom, watching *The Great Escape* or a good Western like *The Good, the Bad, and the Ugly*, she was off on dates. How many dates does it take to meet someone anyway?

Mom would come home and tell Auntie Donna about these guys she was meeting. Some were good, others weren't. Some had potential, and others…well, let's just say they were a complete disaster. Auntie Donna would always tell Mom, "Not everyone is for everyone, but when you find someone who treats you right, hold on to that. Anything less isn't worth your time."

I guess it was hard for Mom, trying to find the right person. But from my perspective, we already had a great life, just the two of us. Why mess with that?

Then one day, everything changed. Mom came home happier than I'd seen her in a long time. She had spent the afternoon at a hot air balloon festival with a man named John, and as she gushed to Auntie Donna about how wonderful the day was, I could feel something shifting. I wasn't thrilled about this "John" guy. Mom seemed happy, but I wasn't feeling warm and fuzzy inside. I wished she'd stop dating altogether.

The following weekend, Mom had another date with John. This time, they spent the day in Philadelphia. And guess where I was? Stuck at home. I'm her support dog—I need to be with her, giving her love and protecting her from harm. Yet, here I was, on the sidelines. When Mom came home, she was glowing as she told Auntie Donna about her day. Uncle Mike, Tigger, Gus, and even the cats didn't seem to care about her date. But me? I cared. I wasn't ready to share my mom.

This pattern of dating continued for months. Every time Mom went out with John, she came home happy. She seemed lighter, more joyful, and full of energy. Then one day, Mom told Auntie Donna that she wanted John to come over for dinner and meet everyone. I thought, "Finally! I'll get to see who this guy is and figure out if he's good enough for Mom." I had my concerns—what if he didn't like me? What if I didn't like him?

Tigger told me to relax. "It's just a dude," he said.

Now, Tigger is pretty protective of his space, and I was half-expecting him to snap at John the moment he walked through the door. Gus, on the other hand, loves everyone. He was already chill about the whole thing.

The day came, and I was nervous. There was a knock at the door, and Tigger, Gus, and I ran to greet the visitor. Mom opened the door, and there he was— the Dude. John stepped inside, and Tigger rushed up to him. I held my breath, waiting for Tigger to snap, but he didn't. Instead, Tigger introduced himself like John had been part of his life all along. I couldn't believe it.

I looked at Tigger in disbelief. "What the heck, Dude?" I asked.

Tigger just shrugged. "He's a good dude."

Gus strolled by, as relaxed as ever. "Yeah, he's cool. Chill out, Remi."

Then it was my turn. Mom introduced me to the Dude, and I was polite but kept my distance. I wasn't ready to trust him yet. I stayed close to Mom the whole night, keeping a watchful eye on John to see if he was hiding anything.

The evening was a blur of laughter and conversation. Mom, Auntie Donna, Uncle Mike, and John sat around the table, enjoying dinner and sharing stories. Everyone seemed to be having a great time. Gus, Tigger, the cats, and I were all hanging out in the living room, but I couldn't relax. I watched John closely, waiting for him to slip up, to show some sign that he wasn't the right guy for Mom.

But he didn't. He was nice and polite the entire night. I couldn't find a single thing wrong with him, and believe me, I tried. Eventually, the evening came to an end, and John went home. Mom and Auntie Donna were both happy, saying how well the dinner had gone.

That night, as I lay beside Mom in bed, I thought about everything. John seemed like a good guy, but I still wasn't sure. It had always been just Mom and me, and I wasn't ready to share her yet. But I realized something—if Mom was happy, then I needed to give this Dude a chance. Maybe he wasn't so bad after all.

In the months that followed, John came over more often. He played with Tigger, Gus, and me, and soon enough, I started to warm up to him. He didn't take Mom away from me. In fact, he became part of our little family. He even took us all on walks and hikes, and I could see how much he cared for Mom.

One evening, after another dinner with John, I sat in the living room with Gus and Tigger. "You were right," I said to Tigger. "He's a good dude."

Tigger gave me a smug look. "Told you."

Gus nodded in agreement. "Sometimes you just have to give people a chance, Remi."

And they were right. John wasn't just some random guy taking up Mom's time. He was a good guy, someone who made Mom smile and brought more happiness into our lives. Over time, John went from being "the Dude" to someone much more important.

Eventually, the Dude became my Dad—but not right away.
Over the months and years, as Mom and John dated, I realized I was part of a new journey. We did everything together. I still got to hang out with Mom,

hike, explore, and watch our favorite movies. But now, I also had Dude by my side, and together, we became the perfect team.

Looking back, I'm really glad I gave John a chance. It's easy to be protective and cautious when new people come into your life, but I've learned that when someone makes the people you love happy, they're worth welcoming in.

So, here's my advice: Don't be afraid to let new people in. They might surprise you in the best way possible.

Alright, friends, that's it for now. I'm off to enjoy a cozy night with Mom and Dude, curled up for another movie marathon. Until next time—keep your hearts open, and remember, it's okay to share the ones you love.

# CHAPTER 12
## *DARN*

Things were going well. Life was good. Mom was happy, and yes, Dude was still very much a part of our lives. Surprisingly, Tigger still hadn't snapped at him, which, for me, was a bit of a shocker. Gus, as usual, was scheming his next great escape from the backyard, though Uncle Mike had fortified the fences so well that Gus's dreams were on indefinite hold. Auntie Donna was constantly hunting for the best treats for Tigger, Gus, and me, and, honestly, I had no complaints about that. Life seemed perfect, and as a support dog, nothing made me happier than knowing everyone around me was happy too—it made my job a whole lot easier.

At least, that's what I thought.

One weekend, I overheard Mom and Dude having a conversation that made my ears perk up. They were talking about moving in together, about finding a place where they could be together more often, making things more "official." My heart dropped. Did that mean I'd have to leave the home I've grown to love? Would I be included in this new life they were building together?

Tigger, of course, thought I was being ridiculous. "You're being silly," he told me, brushing off my concerns. Gus, in his usual laid-back way, added, "Yeah, you're definitely overthinking it."

But deep down, I wasn't so sure. This would be my third home, and I liked where I was now. Everything I needed was here—the familiar smells, the cozy corners, the backyard I loved to explore, and, of course, Uncle Mike, Auntie Donna, Tigger, Gus, and even the two cats (who still didn't make much sense to me). The thought of moving away from all of this filled me with sadness. Why couldn't Dude just move into our house? Why did it have to be somewhere else?

As time passed, my worries grew. Mom and Dude started taking me along on house-hunting trips, and each new house we visited only made me feel more uneasy. None of them had the backyard I loved so much, and none of them felt like home. The layouts were different, the smells unfamiliar, and nothing made me feel comfortable or at ease. With each house, I'd walk in, give it a sniff, and quickly realize it wasn't for me. But Mom and Dude didn't seem to notice my discomfort; they were too busy trying to find the "perfect" place.

After a long day of house hunting, I curled up on the couch, listening as Mom and Dude talked about their frustrations. Apparently, none of the houses they had seen were right for them either. Some were too small, others needed too much work, and some were just too far from where they wanted to live. I sighed with relief, thinking that maybe, just maybe, they'd give up on the idea of moving and stay right where we were. I liked this house. I liked this life. I didn't want anything to change.

Tigger, ever the realist, told me I was delusional. "You're in denial, Remi," he said, as if he could see right through me. Gus, lounging nearby, nodded in agreement. Still, I held onto hope that things would stay the same.

For a while, it seemed like my worries were for nothing. The house hunting slowed down, and Mom and Dude shifted their focus to enjoying the weekends together instead of stressing over finding a new home. We went on more walks, had more cozy movie nights, and life felt back to normal. I thought I had won. Maybe, just maybe, we'd stay in this house forever. I was safe... or so I thought.

Then, one evening, after weeks of peace, the conversation about moving came up again. Mom and Dude sat at the kitchen table, their faces lit up as they excitedly discussed a new house they had seen that day. My ears perked up immediately. Apparently, they had found something they both really liked—a house big enough for all of us, with a backyard, close to Auntie Donna and Uncle Mike, and not too far from my brother Colt, Grandma, and Papa. They were overjoyed, and as much as I wanted to stay in denial, I knew this was it. They weren't giving up this time.

I spent the next few days in quiet anxiety. The thought of leaving everything I loved—Uncle Mike's morning patrols, Auntie Donna's treats, Tigger's grumbles, and Gus's endless escape schemes—made me feel like I was about to lose something precious. I had already lost my real mom when I was adopted, and while I loved my life now, the idea of moving felt like another loss I wasn't ready for.

Mom and Dude took me to see the new house, and just like the others, it didn't feel right to me. Sure, it had a backyard, but it wasn't *my* backyard. The smells were different, the layout unfamiliar, and it didn't give me the comfort I needed. I tried to act uninterested, hoping Mom would notice, but she seemed so thrilled. I knew this meant a lot to her, so I did what I do best—I put on a brave face, wagged my tail, and pretended everything was fine.

The day they decided to buy the house, I sat quietly in the living room, watching as they celebrated. I knew change was coming, and I didn't like it. But I also knew that Mom was happy, and that was what mattered most. As her support dog, my job was to be there for her, even if it meant dealing with changes, I wasn't ready for.

The following weeks were a blur of packing, planning, and preparation. Boxes started piling up, and the impending move loomed over me like a dark cloud. Every time I watched Mom pack, my heart sank a little more. I'd curl up in my favorite spot on the couch, soaking in every last bit of comfort from the home I loved so much.

On the day of the move, I was a bundle of nerves. I stayed close to Mom, trying to be brave as we left the house behind. The new house was everything Mom had wanted—big, spacious, with a backyard that I was sure I'd grow to love—but at that moment, it still felt foreign and strange.

The first night in the new house was rough. I paced around, sniffing everything, trying to get comfortable. Mom, sensing my unease, gave me extra belly rubs and snuggles. Slowly but surely, I began to realize something important: as long as I had Mom, everything would be okay. I didn't need the old backyard, the familiar corners, or even Uncle Mike's morning patrols to feel at home. What made home special wasn't the house—it was the people (and dogs) I loved.

Over time, the new house started to feel more familiar. I found new cozy spots to curl up in, and the backyard—while different—became a place I enjoyed exploring. Tigger and Gus settled in too, and soon enough, life started to feel good again.

Change had come, but I had to trust that no matter where we went, home would always be where we were together. Because in the end, home isn't a place—it's a feeling.

Looking back, I realized that change is hard, but it's not always bad. Sometimes, you just have to take a deep breath, let go of the past, and embrace the new adventure ahead. After all, home isn't just a place—it's where your heart is, and my heart will always be with Mom, no matter where we are.

"Darn it," I thought at first, when I realized my life was about to change. But now, I know it's all part of the journey, and I'm ready to face it, one paw at a time.

Alright, I've got to go now—there's still plenty of unpacking to do!

Later!

# CHAPTER 13
## *PURPOSE*

So, we moved and settled into our new home. But if I'm being honest, it didn't feel right. Everything was upside down, and my usual routines were completely thrown off. I couldn't eat, I couldn't sleep, and no matter how much Mom and Dude (yes, I call him Dude now) tried to snap me out of it, I just wasn't feeling it.

The problem was simple: I missed home.

I was homesick for everything and everyone I'd left behind—the familiar smells, the warmth of Uncle Mike's bed where the "Rat Pack" (Tigger, Gus, and me) would climb in and fall asleep. I missed Auntie Donna's treats, the constant buzz of activity, even the cats with their mysterious ways. And now, here I was in a quiet house, just me, Mom, and Dude. It was strange, unfamiliar, and I couldn't shake the sadness. Everything felt wrong.

Days turned into weeks, and despite their efforts, I still felt off. My appetite was gone, and I spent most of my time just lying around, trying to make sense of it all. I didn't realize it at the time, but things were about to change for me in ways I could never have imagined.

One day, while I was curled up on the couch, half-listening, I overheard Mom and Dude talking about me. They were concerned. Mom was worried that I wasn't adjusting well, and Dude mentioned something about needing more obedience training, that it would help me adjust, socialize with other dogs, and become more confident.

Dude volunteered to take on the task. He said he'd help me become more obedient and focused. At the time, I wasn't exactly thrilled with the idea. I didn't think I needed training—I just needed my old life back. But, as it turned out, Dude had a plan, and that plan changed everything for me.

The very next day, Dude took me on a long walk-through a nearby park. It was a beautiful place, full of trees, streams, and a big pond. You'd think we'd stop and enjoy it, but nope—not even once. This Dude had a mission. It wasn't just a casual stroll; it was serious business. He made me walk beside him, never pulling ahead, never lagging behind, and every few steps, he'd make me stop and sit. We must've walked for three miles, and I probably sat more times that day than I had in my entire life.

At first, I resisted. I'd never had to walk with such precision before. But gradually, something started to shift. The walks became easier, and I began to feel something I hadn't felt in a long time—a sense of purpose. This wasn't just about walking anymore. For every step Dude took, I was right there beside him, and when he stopped at a crosswalk or an intersection, I sat down without hesitation. It was like we were in sync, moving with intention, and that made me feel important.

At first, I'd get nervous when other dogs passed by. I'd jump a little, feeling unsure. But over time, I learned to stay calm. Dude was my leader, and I trusted him. Slowly, I forgot about my worries, about the new house, about the unfamiliar surroundings. Each walk became a little easier, a little more exciting. Every morning, we'd go out, and the day would start with a purpose—a walk where I knew what was expected of me, where I knew my place, and I started feeling more and more like myself again.

I began to look forward to our morning walks. I wasn't just lounging around the house anymore, feeling lost. I had a job to do, a reason to be active. And with each passing day, I grew stronger, more confident in my role. Eventually, Dude took me to an open field, where I could run freely, the wind hitting my face as I sprinted through the tall grass. I'd run so fast, then flop down in the grass, letting it cool me off. It felt amazing, like I had found a new version of freedom.

When Dude called me, I'd come running, eager for the next adventure. I didn't realize it at first but having him as my leader gave me more confidence in myself. I was no longer just a dog trying to adjust to a new home—I was part of something bigger. I had purpose, direction, and it felt good.

One day, Mom joined us on our walk. I was eager to show off my new skills, and as we walked, I made sure to stay right beside Dude, stopping and sitting on command like I'd been doing this forever. Mom was impressed, and for the first time in a while, I felt proud of myself. She smiled and praised me, and I could see the pride in her eyes. That's when it hit me—I wasn't just

Mom's support dog anymore. I was growing, evolving, becoming better, and helping her in new ways.

The months that followed were transformative. I was no longer anxious or homesick. I had fully embraced the new routine, and it wasn't just the training that had changed me—it was the sense of purpose I found in it. Dude had unknowingly taught me that I was capable of so much more than just lounging around or offering comfort. I could lead, I could follow, I could adapt, and most importantly, I could grow.

But what really surprised me was how much happier I felt. I realized that in my old life, things had been easy—almost too easy. I didn't have to think much about what I was doing; I just followed the familiar routine. But now, in this new chapter, I had been given the chance to challenge myself, to learn, and to prove to myself that I could do more. And that gave me a deeper sense of satisfaction than I ever expected.

I started noticing changes in Mom, too. She seemed more at ease, less worried about how I was adjusting. We had settled into our new home, and I was starting to feel like this place wasn't just a house—it was home. Mom and Dude were happy, and that made me happy too. Our walks became longer, more adventurous, and soon, I was exploring places I never thought I'd see.

One day, during one of our morning walks, Dude stopped at the edge of the pond and looked out over the water. I sat down beside him, waiting for the next command, but he didn't say anything. Instead, he looked down at me and smiled. "You've come a long way, Remi," he said quietly. "You've got a lot more in you than you think."

That moment stuck with me. It was true—I had come a long way. I had gone from being a dog lost in his own sadness to becoming a support dog with renewed purpose. I wasn't just helping Mom anymore; I was learning to help myself. And with that, I realized something important: Purpose isn't just about having a job to do. It's about finding meaning in the everyday, in the small things, in the moments when you push yourself just a little further than you thought you could.

Life wasn't about lounging on the couch or sticking to the familiar routine anymore. It was about walking with intention, learning new things, and growing—both for myself and for the people I love.

Looking back now, I understand that the move wasn't the end of something—it was the beginning of something new. I didn't lose my old life; I gained a new one, one where I was more confident, more capable, and more in tune with the world around me.

I also learned that sometimes, you have to step outside your comfort zone to find your true purpose. It's not always easy, but when you do, you realize just how strong and capable you really are.

So, if you're ever feeling lost or out of place, remember this: It's okay to be unsure at first. But with time, patience, and a little guidance, you'll find your way. You'll find your purpose.

And who knows? You might even find that you're capable of more than you ever imagined.

Alright, friends, that's all for now. I'm off to take another adventure with Mom and Dude. Remember, no matter where life takes you, find your purpose, and embrace it fully. You'll be amazed at what you can achieve.

# CHAPTER 14
## *THE DOG SHOW*

Mom and Dude were talking about going away for the weekend, and then they both looked at me and said, "What about Remi?" What about me? I thought to myself. After all the training and hard work, I've put in as a support dog, isn't the whole point to be with them all the time? A bit annoyed, I started to think that all my efforts were going unnoticed. I mean, I've come a long way, Dude—learning to handle myself in almost every situation, though I still get rattled around other dogs, mean people, and those old loud cars. But no one's perfect, right?

I couldn't bear to listen any longer, so I walked away from their conversation. I found my bed, curled up, and pretended to sleep, but inside, I was fuming. I couldn't believe it. This Dude had come into our lives, moved me away from everything familiar, and now they were planning a trip without me. What did I do wrong?

As I lay there, I heard Mom's voice call, "Remi." I figured they'd had a change of heart, so I ran back to find her. She smiled and said, "Hey Remi! Do you want to spend the weekend with Auntie Donna and Uncle Mike? Tigger, Gus, and your brother Colt will all be there!"

Well, of course, I did! I wagged my tail with excitement and ran straight to the door, ready to go. Who needed their weekend getaway? My weekend with my family was going to be way better!

We arrived at Auntie Donna and Uncle Mike's house, and I couldn't wait to see everyone. The moment Mom opened the car door, I jumped out and darted toward the house. Auntie Donna opened the door, and I rushed in like I owned the place, feeling great… until I ran into Tigger. *Whelp.* I had forgotten who the presumed alpha was around here—Tigger. He's always a little snappy about his space, so I calmed myself down.

I greeted Gus, but as usual, he wanted to go outside immediately. It seemed like nothing had changed—his 15 minutes were up, and he needed to relieve himself. I heard Mom calling goodbye, but I was already halfway out to the backyard with Tigger and Gus, eager to share all my new adventures.

As we wandered outside, I told them all about my training and how Dude had taught me to walk properly and sit on command.

Gus, always laid back, gave me a confused look. "You learned how to walk and sit? Can't you do that on your own? Is Dude training you for the National Dog Show or something?"

I blinked, "What's the National Dog Show?"

"The National Dog Show," Gus explained, "is where dogs show off their skills—walking, sitting, climbing, doing tricks like rolling over, jumping through hoops, all that fancy stuff. Don't you remember Auntie Donna and your mom watching it on TV every year?"

"Oh," I said, realizing that I might have seen it before but never paid attention.

Tigger chimed in, "Remi, Dude is a professional dog trainer. They're probably getting you ready for the National Dog Show."

"No way!" I exclaimed, feeling a mix of disbelief and panic. I hadn't signed up for that! I was fine being a support dog and learning obedience, but the National Dog Show? That was way beyond what I thought I was capable of.

Then I remembered something Dude had once said during one of our long walks. We had stopped by the pond, and he'd looked out over the water. I sat beside him, waiting for the next command, but he hadn't said anything. Instead, he looked down at me and smiled, "You've come a long way, Remi. You've got a lot more in you than you think."

Now, I realized what he meant—he saw potential in me that I hadn't yet seen in myself.

Just then, my brother Colt arrived, and of course, Tigger couldn't keep quiet. He told Colt everything, and they all started laughing at me. Feeling embarrassed, I walked over to the patio door, wanting to go inside and get away from their teasing. I needed time to think. Was this all true? Was I really being trained for something as big as the National Dog Show?

As the afternoon went on, Tigger and Gus kept smirking and making comments about my "future stardom." But Colt, ever the wise and steady brother, pulled me aside. "Little brother, don't let them get to you. If you do end up at the National Dog Show, those two will be jealous because you've done something they haven't. But even if you don't, remember, you're doing great, and I'm proud of you. Our birth mom would be too. Relax and embrace whatever adventures come your way. You never know where they might lead."

Colt doesn't say much, but when he does, it's always worth listening to. His words calmed me down, and I started to see things differently. Maybe all this training wasn't just about obedience—it could be about something bigger, about growing into the best version of myself. And if that meant taking on new challenges, then so be it.

Colt and I sat together for a while, and he reminded me that being trained to be a better support dog was a good thing. "Change is good," he said. "It means you're growing. Not everyone gets the chance to grow like you have, Remi. That's why some people—or dogs—get jealous instead of being happy for others. But you're doing great, and we're all proud of you, even if we like giving you a hard time."

By the end of the weekend, Gus and Tigger had stopped teasing me as much, mostly because I had learned to ignore them. When Sunday came and Mom and Dude arrived to pick me up after their weekend away, I was ready to go home, feeling more at peace. Sure, the idea of competing in a National Dog Show still seemed overwhelming, but I realized that, whatever came my way, I'd be ready for it. I was growing, learning, and finding new ways to be useful, and that felt good.

Whether I end up in a show or just continue being the best support dog I can be, I know one thing for sure: I've got a lot more in me than I ever thought possible. And that's something to be proud of.

As we headed home, I snuggled into the backseat, feeling at peace with whatever the future held. I realized that sometimes, we just have to embrace the unknown and trust that we're on the right path.

So, the National Dog Show? Who knows. But for now, I'm happy just being me—Remi, the support dog with a little more purpose every day.

Remember, peace comes from embracing the journey, not worrying about where it will take you. I'm off to enjoy some belly rubs and relax after a fun weekend.

# CHAPTER 15
## *UNWANTED COMPANY*

The mornings had become routine, almost clockwork. Dude would get up, and as soon as he was ready, he'd come over to my bed, pat me on the head, and slip on my collar. We'd head out the door for our morning walk. But first, like any good dog, I had to take care of my "business." It was a simple process: sniff around, find the right spot, and get things done.

Except lately, it wasn't that simple. Every morning, without fail, Daisy—the neighbor's dog—would come bounding toward me before I could even start. Like, seriously, girl? Can't a dog have a little privacy? Every single morning, she'd charge over, all excited, tail wagging, as if we were best friends. But honestly, I wasn't interested in making new friends. I had my family, my routine, and my world. I didn't need Daisy pushing her way into it.

As usual, Dude exchanged a few words with Daisy's owner while I stood there, trying to focus on my business. But there was Daisy, bouncing around like it was the best day of her life. I wasn't having it.

I looked up at Dude, silently pleading for him to get us moving. Fortunately, he seemed to pick up on my discomfort, giving me a gentle nudge. Finally, we were off on our walk. I glanced back quickly to see if Daisy was still watching, and sure enough, she was sitting there, staring as if waiting for me to come back. I rolled my eyes and trotted on, trying to shake off the irritation.

The walk felt better. I focused on the familiar rhythm of our routine—left, right, stop, sit—it was comforting. I liked having that sense of purpose with Dude by my side. The world was peaceful during those early morning walks. The air was fresh, the trees swayed gently, and the sound of our footsteps filled the quiet streets.

But I couldn't shake the nagging feeling that Daisy was still watching me. That she was somehow part of my world now. Ugh. I didn't want to make new friends.

A few days later, it happened again. We were barely out the door when Daisy came running over, her excitement overwhelming as usual. This time, though, she was even more persistent. She didn't just watch from a distance—she tried to walk with us.

I did my best to ignore her, to pretend she wasn't there, but she trotted alongside me, panting, her eyes gleaming with excitement. I sped up, hoping she'd get the hint, but she kept pace.

"Remi, don't be rude," Dude said with a chuckle, noticing my frustration. "Daisy just wants to be your friend."

Friend? I didn't need another friend. Especially one like Daisy, who didn't seem to understand the concept of personal space. I sighed, resigned to the fact that she wasn't going anywhere.

Over the next week, it became obvious that Daisy wasn't going to give up. Every morning, like clockwork, she'd bounce over, tail wagging, ready to disrupt our peaceful routine. No matter how much I tried to ignore her, she was relentless. I couldn't understand why she kept coming back. Couldn't she see I wasn't interested? Didn't she know I had

important things to do, like training for the National Dog Show?

But after a while, something began to shift in me. I started to wonder why she kept coming back. What was it about me that made her so eager to be my friend?

One morning, after yet another awkward interaction with Daisy, Dude and I continued our walk as usual. But this time, something felt different. As we walked through the quiet streets, I couldn't help but think about Daisy's persistence. Every day, she showed up, full of energy and excitement, even when I ignored her or made it clear I wasn't interested. She never gave up, always hoping for a connection.

It hit me then—Daisy wasn't just being annoying. She was showing me something I hadn't seen before. While I was stuck in my routine, comfortable with my small circle of family and friends, she was open to the world, eager to make new connections and experience new things. Her enthusiasm, though overwhelming, came from a place of genuine joy and curiosity.

"Maybe I've been too closed off," I thought. Maybe I'd been so focused on maintaining my routine and my comfort zone that I hadn't allowed myself the chance to open up to new experiences—or new friends.

The next day, as we headed out for our walk, I found myself glancing around, wondering when Daisy would appear. Sure enough, there she was, sprinting toward me with her usual uncontainable excitement. This time, though, I didn't bristle at her presence. Instead, I gave her a small wag of my tail. It wasn't much, but it was a start.

"Morning, Daisy," I said, a little reluctantly.

Daisy noticed immediately. Her tail wagged even harder, like she'd just hit the jackpot. She trotted beside me, and for the first time, I didn't speed up to avoid her. I let her walk with us. I still kept a little distance, but I didn't mind her as much as I had before.

"Good morning, Remi!" Daisy chirped, her enthusiasm bubbling over. "Are you going for your daily walk?"

"Yes, we are," I responded, trying to sound neutral.

"That's wonderful! I hope it's a beautiful walk today!" she added, her voice full of joy.

I hesitated for a moment, then replied, "Thank you, and you have a wonderful day yourself, Daisy."

As the days passed, things began to change. I stopped avoiding Daisy, and I even found myself looking forward to seeing her in the mornings. She wasn't so bad after all. Sure, she was pushy and a little too enthusiastic for my taste, but her heart was in the right place. Slowly, without realizing it, I started to enjoy her company.

One morning, as we walked together, side by side, I realized something important: maybe there was more to life than sticking to the familiar. Maybe there was something to be gained from letting others in, from opening up to new friendships and experiences.

Daisy had taught me something I hadn't expected—sometimes, the best things in life come from unexpected places. I had been so focused on keeping things the way they were, safely within my comfort zone, that I almost missed out on something good—something joyful.

Our walks continued, and I found myself relaxing more, enjoying the world around me in a new way. I even caught myself running with Daisy a few times, letting loose, forgetting about all the things that used to bother me. It felt good. It felt freeing.

One morning, after we finished our walk, Dude bent down and gave me a pat on the head. "You've changed, Remi," he said with a smile. "You're more open, more at peace."

And he was right. I had changed. I had found peace, not by sticking to the routine, but by letting go of my resistance, accepting new things, and allowing myself to be open to what life had to offer—whether it was a new friend like Daisy or just the simple joy of a morning walk.

As we headed back home, Daisy bounced away to her own yard, and I watched her go with a feeling of contentment. I was glad she hadn't given up on me. Glad she had been persistent enough to break through my walls.

Life, I realized, isn't just about routines or sticking to what you know. It's about embracing the unexpected, welcoming new friends, and finding joy in things that once made you uncomfortable.

Daisy taught me that sometimes, the peace we seek doesn't come from shutting out the world, but from opening ourselves up to it. And when we do, we find that the world has so much more to offer than we ever imagined.

So, the next time you find yourself resisting change or pushing something new away, remember this: peace isn't about keeping things the same. It's about accepting life as it comes, with all its surprises, challenges, and yes, even the Daisies of the world.

Alright, friends, that's it for now. I'm off to enjoy another peaceful walk with Dude—and maybe even Daisy. Until next time, keep your hearts open, and don't be afraid to let in a little unexpected joy.

# CHAPTER 16
## *FINDING DAD*

Life had settled into a comfortable rhythm in my new home. I had found my new purpose, and things were going well. Even my training had intensified. Every morning, Dude and I would go on a three-mile walk, during which I'd take in the fresh morning air, hear the birds chirping, and feel the dew on the grass under my paws. As the sun rose over the East Coast, the world around me felt alive, vibrant, and full of possibility. It was one of my favorite parts of the day, where I could clear my mind and prepare for whatever lay ahead.

In the evenings, our routine changed. Dude and I would head to the local park for more intense training sessions. The park became our little training ground, where we worked on skills I never knew I had. Dude started slowly with basic commands like "sit" and "stay," but as time went on, I learned how to hold a position for my own safety. I learned how to jump onto walls and balance on them, walk across narrow surfaces, and even climb logs that were two feet off the ground. Dude believed I had more in me than I thought, and every evening he pushed me to do better, to go higher, to try harder.

At first, I wasn't so sure of myself. Jumping off logs, scaling obstacles—it was all so new. But Dude was always there, encouraging me. His words gave me confidence: "You've got this, Remi. I know you can do it." And with his support, I started to believe in myself. Eventually, I could jump, climb, and balance without hesitation. The best part was hearing

Dude's voice say, "Good job, Remi," every time I nailed a trick.

I also started learning new words like "down," "up," "shake a paw," "hug," "jump," "walk," "roll over," and "lay down." Each word came with a task, and while I wasn't a huge fan of the "roll over" command, I really liked the one for "hug." That was an easy one—I'd wrap my paws around Dude, and he'd laugh every time. It felt good to see him happy.

Dude even created an obstacle course at the park, using the natural environment to challenge me. I got better and better as we trained, and pretty soon, people started watching us with amazement. I overheard them talking about how impressed they were with my skills. It felt great to be recognized for all the hard work I'd been putting in.

One day, Dude invited Mom to come watch one of our evening training sessions. I was excited to show her everything I had learned. As we began, Mom watched from the sidelines, her eyes wide with pride as she said, "Remi, you're such a good boy!"

Dude decided to show off one of my more impressive tricks. "Remi, up!" he called out. Without missing a beat, I leaped onto a log, balancing myself like a tightrope walker. I could hear Mom gasp in amazement.

But things took a turn when Dude gave the next command. "Remi, down," he said, signaling for me to jump off the log. As I launched myself into the air, I heard Mom cry out, "Oh my, no, Remi!"

Wait, what? What did she mean, "no"? I was already committed to the jump, and here was my mom, telling me to stop mid-air. There was no stopping now. I landed the jump perfectly and sat beside Dude, confused by her reaction.

Dude gently explained to Mom, "Never express fear when Remi's performing a trick. He can sense your emotions. We need to show confidence, so he feels comfortable while he's doing these things."

Mom nodded, understanding that while she loved me dearly and was only concerned for my safety, it was important for her to stay calm. After all, I wasn't just a support dog anymore—I was learning new skills, maybe even for the National Dog Show! These tricks weren't dangerous—they were exciting challenges, and with Dude guiding me, I knew I was safe. Slowly but surely, Mom started to see that too, realizing that what we were doing wasn't risky; it was fun and rewarding for both of us.

For the next hour, Dude continued showing Mom the various tricks I'd learned, and soon enough, she was cheering me on, full of confidence. It felt great knowing that both Dude and Mom believed in me.

As we were wrapping up, a stranger approached us. He had been watching our training session and seemed impressed. "Wow, your dog is amazing," he said to Dude. "Do you train other dogs? Could you train mine?"

Dude chuckled. "No, I'm not really interested in that," he said.

The man was persistent. "How did you learn to train dogs like this?" he asked.

Dude shrugged and explained, "I grew up with German Shepherds. I was responsible for training them, and I guess it stuck."

The stranger nodded, clearly grateful for the tips Dude shared with him about starting with basic commands like "sit" and leading with confidence. He thanked Dude and walked away, leaving me feeling a little puffed up with pride.

Then something happened that completely threw me off. Mom turned to Dude and said, "I'm so impressed with the both of you. Thank you, Daddy, for training Remi."

Wait. What? *Daddy?* I froze for a moment. Did I hear that right? I thought I had been calling this guy "Dude" all this time, but now he's *Daddy?* Confused, I tried to shake off the feeling, but then Mom said it again, "Daddy."

I looked at Dude—no, *Daddy*—and started to replay everything in my head. When did he go from being Dude to Dad? I had always thought of him as just the guy who came into our lives, took me on long walks, and trained me. But as we walked home that evening, something clicked.

I thought about all the time we had spent together. All those mornings when he woke up early to take me on walks. All those moments when he encouraged me to do better, to believe in myself, to push my limits. I remembered the times I failed during training, and how he was always there, right by my side, never disappointed—just patient, offering me another chance to try again.

Then I remembered that day by the pond, when Dude—no, Dad—looked at me and smiled, saying, "You've come a long way, Remi. You've got a lot more in you than you think."

Suddenly, it all made sense. I had never known my real dad, and I hadn't really thought much about it before. But now, I realized that Dude had become more than just a trainer or someone who happened to be with my mom. He had been there for me in every way that mattered, encouraging me, supporting me, and believing in me, even when I didn't believe in myself.

That night, as Mom and Dad got ready for bed, I jumped up on the bed and curled up between them. I listened as Mom told Dad how proud she was of me and how much I'd accomplished. I felt a warmth in my heart, knowing that we were a family—Mom, Dad, and me.

I had never called him Dad before, but in my heart, I knew that's exactly who he was.

The next morning, our routine was the same, but it felt different. As we walked through the park, I felt an even stronger connection to the man I once thought of as just "Dude." Now, he was my Dad, and that realization made me feel even more secure, more loved, and more determined to keep growing, keep learning, and keep pushing myself.

As we passed by the pond, Dad looked down at me again and said, "You've come so far, Remi. And I know you've still got so much more ahead of you."

And for the first time, I fully believed him.

That night, as I curled up in bed, sandwiched between Mom and Dad, I knew that I had found more than just a home—I had found my family.

Dude was more than just a guy who trained me and took me on long walks. He was my dad. And together with Mom, we were the family I never knew I needed.

Life was good. I had a purpose, I had love, and most importantly, I had peace knowing that no matter what challenges came my way, I had my family by my side, cheering me on every step of the way.

And that's all a dog like me could ever ask for.

# CHAPTER 17
## *GROOMING DAY*

It was a Monday, and I was super excited to see Tigger, Gus, Auntie Donna, and Uncle Mike. But it was also that time of the month—grooming day. As I leaped into the back of Mom's car, we started our journey, and I couldn't help but feel the rush of excitement. Grooming days were always an adventure. The car ride itself was amazing—Mom had her music on full blast, singing at the top of her lungs, missing almost every beat, but it didn't matter. She was happy, and that made me happy. Her joy made the world feel bright, and I was more alive than ever, full of energy and purpose, all thanks to Dad and the training he'd been putting me through.

As I sat there, watching the trees blur by, the sun beaming through the gaps in the forest and touching my face, I couldn't help but reflect on my journey. I realized something important: you can't connect the dots looking forward, only looking backward. You have to trust that somehow; the dots will connect in your future. Change was tough, but looking back, it had all been good for me.

When we finally arrived at Auntie Donna and Uncle Mike's house, the Groomer Lady was already there with her big van parked out front, proudly advertising "Mobile Pet Spa" on the side. Fancy, right? This wasn't just any grooming experience—this was a full-on spa day, and boy, I needed it. Auntie Donna greeted us at the door and said to Mom,

"Gus is finishing up, and Tigger's already done. He's inside lounging on the couch."

Mom smiled and turned to me. "Remi, you're next!"

Gus was leaving the Mobile Pet Spa as I waited my turn, and he couldn't resist poking fun. "Getting groomed for the National Dog Show, huh?"

Wait, what? National Dog Show? Was all my training with Dad leading up to something big like that? My heart raced with excitement. I leaped into the truck like I had a purpose, eager to look my best. I hopped up onto the bath bed, ready for my spa treatment. My nails were clipped, my hair was trimmed to perfection, and as the water drenched my fur, the Lady Groomer lathered me up with the most delightful-smelling soap. Did I mention how much I love spa days? Especially now that I was preparing for my "big day," whatever that might be.

An hour later, I was done, looking and feeling like a brand-new dog. I strutted out into the backyard, my fur gleaming in the sunlight, feeling fresh and clean. Tigger and Gus spotted me immediately as they ran circles around the yard, chasing each other's tails. They both rushed over, and Gus couldn't resist teasing me again.

"Remi, are you ready for your big day?" Gus asked with a mischievous grin.

Playing it cool, I replied, "What big day?"

Tigger jumped in. "You know, the National Dog Show!"

I tried to shrug it off. "I don't know if that's happening," I said, trying to keep my excitement in check. I mean, sure,

all the training made sense now, but I hadn't heard anything official from Mom or Dad.

Gus, always the instigator, grinned. "That's why you got groomed today. For the show!"

I was unsure, but I didn't want to crush their excitement. "We'll see what happens," I said, leaving the possibility open. After all, it was kind of thrilling to think about.

Just then, I overheard Auntie Donna talking to Mom. "Remi looks so handsome. With all the training he's had, he'd do great in the National Dog Show," she said.

My ears perked up. Was it really happening? Could this be true?

Mom smiled but shook her head. "He does look great, but Remi can't compete."

I froze. What? Why not?

Mom continued, "Remi doesn't have his breeding certificate, which disqualifies him from entering the National Dog Show."

My heart sank. All that excitement, all those thoughts of performing in front of a crowd—gone in an instant. I had been denied because of a technicality. All that training… what was it for?

I glanced over at Tigger and Gus, who were giggling like pups. It hit me— this had all been a prank. They'd been teasing me the whole time, filling my head with the idea of going to the National Dog Show, knowing full well that I couldn't even participate. I barked at them in frustration and flopped down on the grass, feeling disappointed.

Then Uncle Mike came outside, holding an envelope. "A letter came for you, Remi," he said, handing it to Mom.

Mom looked at the envelope and smiled. "I know what this is... Remi, this is for you."

I perked up, my disappointment fading just a little. What now? No more surprises, please—I couldn't handle another rollercoaster of emotions.

Mom opened the letter and started reading it aloud. "Remi is now an officially certified support dog, approved by the government."

Wait, what? Officially certified? I had no idea this was even a thing! I mean, I knew I was a support dog because that's what I do, but being recognized by the government? That was something else entirely.

Meanwhile, Auntie Donna, Uncle Mike, and Mom were all smiling, thrilled with the news. I looked over at Tigger and Gus, and for once, they were speechless. They didn't have that status—official, government-approved support dog status.

I was still coming to terms with everything. I wasn't going to the National Dog Show, but I was being trained for something even more important: to be the best support dog I could be. Sure, it wasn't the glitzy world of shows and trophies, but my role as a support dog carried a deeper purpose, a role that helped people like Mom, who needed me every day.

Tigger and Gus eventually stopped teasing, realizing that what I was doing was something they couldn't fully grasp. Sure, the Dog Show was a glamorous dream, but being a support dog wasn't about glamour—it was about heart, loyalty, and dedication.

As the day went on, I found myself thinking less about the disappointment of not going to the show and more about the honor of what I'd just achieved. I was recognized for my purpose, for the role I played in making my family's life better. And in the end, wasn't that what truly mattered?

Later that day, as we all gathered in the backyard, Auntie Donna brought out treats, and Uncle Mike joined us with his usual humor. The sun began to set, casting a golden glow over the yard. I watched as Tigger and Gus chased each other again, their laughter filling the air. But for the first time, I didn't feel the need to join in. I sat there, quietly content, realizing that my purpose was bigger than any show or competition.

Mom came over and sat beside me, gently petting my head. "You're such a good boy, Remi," she whispered, and I knew she meant it.

And that's when it truly hit me. Life wasn't about winning trophies or being in the spotlight. My role wasn't about recognition or praise. It was about being there for my family, doing my best every day, and fulfilling my purpose as a support dog. That's where my value lay—in the quiet, unseen moments, in the love and care I provided.

The dots that I couldn't connect before now made sense. Every bit of training, every early morning walk, every obstacle I'd overcome, it was all leading me to this—my role, my place, my purpose. I was more than just a dog. I was part of a family, part of something bigger than myself.

As the evening turned into night and we all made our way inside, I felt a deep sense of peace settle over me. Gus and Tigger, with all their teasing, had finally gotten a taste of their own medicine. Sure, I wasn't going to the National Dog Show, but that didn't matter. I had found something far more meaningful—my true purpose.

That night, as I curled up in my bed, I smiled, knowing that I didn't need the validation of a competition. I was enough just as I was. A certified support dog, a loving member of my family, and the happiest dog in the world.

And as I drifted off to sleep, I knew one thing for certain: this was my true purpose.

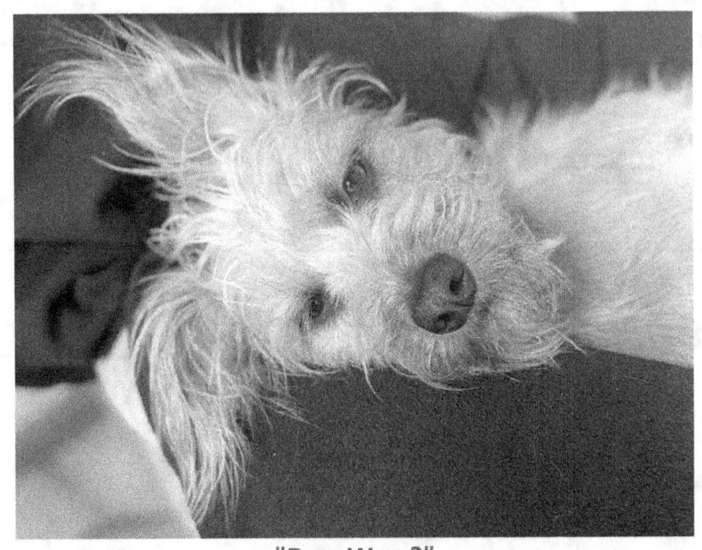

"REMI WALK?"

*"Anybody who doesn't know what soap tastes like never washed a dog."*

– Franklin P. Jones

# CHAPTER 18
## *THE BARBECUE*

It was shaping up to be a perfect day—sun shining, a gentle breeze in the air, and the smell of food cooking on the grill. Today, we were having a big playdate at our home. My brother Colt, my pals Tigger and Gus, and even Daisy were invited to come over. It wasn't just for us dogs either—Mom and Dad had invited family and friends over for a barbecue. I was excited. This wasn't just any ordinary day; it was a day to show off my fresh grooming and to feel the pride of having recently been certified by the government as a Support Dog. It was an honor to wear that badge. It meant I had a purpose and a responsibility, and I took both very seriously.

But beyond the responsibility, I was really looking forward to one particular treat—bacon! Dad always made a special batch for me during these family gatherings, and today, he'd probably make enough for the whole Rat Pack and Daisy too.

As I ran around the yard in the morning, I could see Dad getting everything ready. He'd made sure the barbecue had enough propane, set up extra chairs for everyone, and was already busy grilling. Mom was inside preparing the food—hamburgers, hot dogs, and who knows what else. I took a quick survey of the yard and decided I'd better hide a few bones for safekeeping. Gus had a bad habit of digging up everyone's bones and hiding them in impossible-to-find places. It was his favorite game—taking everyone's treats and burying them for later. Not that anyone was impressed by it.

After a while, I paused to admire Dad's handiwork. The yard looked perfect, ready for company, and as Mom brought out the food, I couldn't help but smile. This was my family, and I loved seeing them so happy.

Then, we heard voices from the gate. My heart leaped with excitement, and I ran over to greet Tigger and Gus as they trotted in with Auntie Donna and Uncle Mike. As soon as Auntie Donna said, "Hi, Remi," I was already off, chasing Tigger and Gus around the yard.

As we ran, Tigger turned to me and said, "I'm proud of you, Remi, for getting your certification."

Tigger was usually the one giving me grief, so hearing that from him made me feel even prouder. Tigger didn't hand out compliments easily.

Gus, ever the jokester, walked over, dropped a bone at my feet, and said, "Yeah, Remi, that's pretty cool. You're all official now."

I was feeling on top of the world, but just then, Daisy arrived, racing over to us, full of energy. "What's going on?" she asked, her tail wagging so hard it looked like it might fly off.

"Tigger was just telling Remi how proud he is that he's certified as a support dog. It's all official now," Gus chimed in.

Daisy's eyes widened. "Wow, Remi, that's amazing! But when are you going to the National Dog Show?"

I looked down at my paws, feeling a mix of pride and uncertainty. Before I could say anything, Gus jumped in. "Remi can't. He's not a purebred. It's a technicality, you know."

A wave of disappointment hit me, but I didn't want to show it. "Yeah, it's a bummer," I muttered.

Then, something unexpected happened—Daisy walked over and kissed me on the cheek. My eyes widened in surprise as Gus and Tigger burst out giggling like pups. I was stunned. I'd never had a girl kiss me before, and now my face felt like it was on fire.

"Hey, guys," Colt's voice broke in as he strolled over.

"What's going on here?"

I was still flustered when Colt asked, "So, is she your girlfriend, Remi?"

"What? No, no!" I stammered, my heart racing.
Daisy giggled and said, "Remi's a good friend," before giving me a wink. I gulped, feeling something tighten inside me that I couldn't quite explain.

Before I could figure out what was going on, Dad called us over. Each of us was handed a strip of bacon. We settled under the big shady tree in the yard, the cool grass beneath us, and the smell of food filling the air. The Rat Pack, Daisy, and I sat together, enjoying the day, talking about our next adventures and all the fun we'd had in the past year.

As we lay there, Tigger started telling the story of Gus's infamous "Great Escape." Gus shook his head and laughed. "If it weren't for Remi, we would've made it," he joked.

Meanwhile, Dad, Uncle Mike, and Papa were working at the far end of the yard, moving things around. Tigger squinted in their direction and asked, "What are they doing?" Colt shrugged, "Not sure."

We didn't pay much attention, though. Being under the cool shade of the tree felt too nice, and we were having a good time, just chatting and relaxing, lost in our stories.

That was until Papa suddenly called out, "Hey, everyone! We have a special show happening today. Let's all gather around over here!"

Our ears perked up, curiosity growing as we wondered what was in store.

I perked up, curious. What show?

Mom called out, "Where's Remi?"

That's when I knew something was up. My ears twitched, and I got to my feet, walking over to where everyone was gathering. People were blocking my view, but I could hear them talking. Grandma asked, "Are we going to see Remi perform today?"

Perform? No one said anything to me about a performance.

The crowd parted, and there, in front of a setup of obstacles—picnic tables, chairs, planks, and even an old playset—stood Dad. My heart skipped a beat. What was going on?

Dad called out, "Remi, come!" Without hesitation, I trotted over, still unsure of what was happening. I looked back at Mom, Uncle Mike, Auntie Donna, Grandma, and Papa. They were all smiling and clapping, clearly excited.

The Rat Pack and Daisy had front-row seats, watching closely. I turned my head to Dad, still puzzled. "Remi and I are going to give everyone a great Dog Show," he announced.

A Dog Show? My heart raced with a mix of nerves and excitement. I hadn't realized we were putting on a show for everyone, but I trusted Dad. He had guided me through so much, always believing in me.

Dad crouched down and gave me that familiar look, the one that always calmed me. "You've come a long way, Remi. You've got a lot more in you than you think. Let's give them a great show."

With that, we began.

The first command came, and just like we had practiced, I moved through the obstacles with precision and focus. We flowed together like a well-rehearsed dance, each command followed by my perfect execution. I jumped, balanced, crawled, and leaped across the obstacles Dad had set up. The crowd cheered with every successful move, and I could hear the excitement building.

At one point, I glanced at the Rat Pack and Daisy. Tigger was grinning, Gus was distracted (probably thinking about stars again), Colt gave me a proud nod, and Daisy… well, Daisy winked at me. That gave me the extra boost I needed to nail the next jump.

As we reached the end of the obstacle course, I heard Mom's voice cheering, "Good boy, Remi!" Dad gave me one last command, and with a final leap, I landed right beside him, the crowd erupting in applause.

Dad bent down, ruffled my fur, and whispered, "You did great, buddy."

The show was over, but the love and pride from everyone made me feel like a champion. I wasn't at the National Dog Show, but I didn't need to be. This was my stage, and I had performed for the people who mattered most.

As the cheers quieted down, Mom came out with a cake, and to my surprise, she also had a special dog-friendly cake for me, the Rat Pack, and Daisy.

Mom said, "We had a great Dog Show today, thanks to Remi, the Support Dog. And since we're all here, we're also celebrating Remi's official certification as a government-approved support dog!"

The clapping started up again, and Papa leaned down to rub my head, saying, "That's a good boy, Remi."

As Mom cut the cake, Dad brought our special cake over to the shady tree. "Here you guys go," he said, smiling at me, Tigger, Gus, Colt, and Daisy. We dug in, each of us finding a spot to sit and enjoy our well-earned treat.

Colt looked up at me between bites. "You know, little brother, that was a very impressive Dog Show. It was better than the National Dog Show."

Gus nodded in agreement. "Yeah, forget about the technicalities. You're the best dog in any show, Remi."

Then, out of nowhere, Daisy came over and gave me a kiss on the cheek. The Rat Pack burst into giggles like a bunch of puppies.

"I told you guys' Daisy was Remi's girlfriend!" Tigger teased, grinning from ear to ear.

I couldn't help but smile, feeling loved and proud. In the end, I got my "Dog Show". Even though I never made it to the National Dog Show because of a "technicality," I wouldn't trade today for anything. This was where I truly belonged, surrounded by the people and dogs that mattered most.

Oh, and remember that bone Gus gave me earlier? I later found out it was one of the bones I'd buried. Figures.

But that didn't matter. Today was perfect.

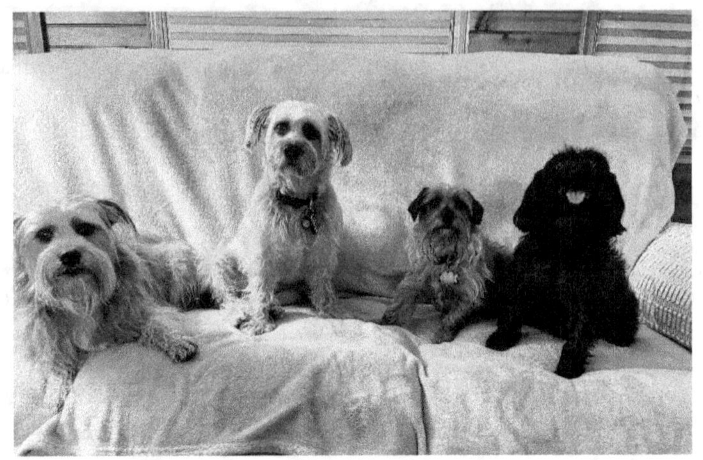



*"A dog is the only thing on earth that loves
you more than you love yourself."*

— Josh Billings

# EPILOGUE
## *THE TAIL END OF THE JOURNEY*

As I sit here reflecting on everything that has happened, I can't help but feel grateful for this incredible journey. Every bark, every wag, every leap over a hurdle—it's all led me to this moment, surrounded by love, warmth, and the certainty that I have found my place in the world.

Life is full of unexpected twists and turns. At times, I didn't know what was coming next. From being adopted, leaving behind the home I knew, and adjusting to new routines, to finding my role as a support dog, it was a path filled with uncertainty. But through it all, there was one constant: love. The love of my family, friends, and even the new people I met along the way who helped shape me into the dog I am today.

When I first joined my mom and met Dude—who later became my Dad— I had no idea where life would take me. At times, the changes were tough, but as I look back, I can see how each step led me to a deeper sense of purpose. Every new skill I learned, every challenge I faced, helped me grow not just as a dog, but as a companion, a guide, and a friend. I realized that even when life throws you into situations you weren't prepared for, you can always find your footing if you trust the process, trust yourself, and trust the people around you.

The world is a big place, full of different smells, sounds, and sights. At first, it can seem overwhelming—kind of like my training sessions with Dad. He believed I could do more, pushed me to new limits, and always encouraged me when I doubted myself. I didn't think I could jump on walls, balance on logs, or stay calm in busy parks, but slowly, I did. Little by little, I began to realize that there's always more strength inside you than you think. Sometimes, you just need the right nudge (or a loving Dad) to help you unlock it.

But beyond the tricks and training, the biggest lesson I learned was something more profound. Life isn't about mastering obstacles; it's about the connections you make along the way. It's about being there for others, offering a comforting nuzzle when someone is sad or a joyful bark when there's something to celebrate. It's about showing up with all the love you have and giving it freely. That's what makes a difference—not just for those around you, but for yourself too.

## Happiness in the Small Moments

I want to share something important with you, something I learned through this journey: happiness isn't found in achieving great feats or being the best at something. Sure, I trained hard, and yes, I even did a dog show in my backyard that made my family proud. But the real joy came in the quieter moments—the mornings when the sun warmed my fur as I lay under the tree, the gentle pats on the head from Dad after a successful walk, and the way Mom's voice always softened when she said, "Good boy, Remi."

Happiness, I've come to realize, was never about winning or showing off. It was about the journey—the everyday walks, the belly rubs, and the simple presence of the people (and dogs) who love you. It was in discovering who I was, not by comparing myself to others, but by embracing who I am.

I wasn't meant to be a show dog, and that's okay. My purpose was something even greater: to be there for my family, to support them, and to bring joy to their lives in ways I never imagined. That's what I hope for you too— that you find your purpose and realize that happiness is not a destination but the way you walk your path.

## The Power of Purpose

Being a certified support dog is an honor, but more than that, it's a privilege. Every time I sit beside Mom, every time I give her a nuzzle when she's feeling down, or walk with her to lift her spirits, I feel a sense of fulfillment. It's not about the title or the recognition—it's about knowing that I am here for her, helping her navigate life's ups and downs. And as much as I support her, she supports me. That's the beauty of love—it's always a two-way street.

We all need someone to lean on, whether you're a dog or a human. And sometimes, we don't even realize how much we need each other until we're there, shoulder to shoulder (or in my case, paw to knee), walking through life together. That's what gives life meaning—being present for the people we love and knowing they're there for us in return.

## For Those Reading My Story

Thank you for reading my story, I hope it brings you a little comfort and joy. Life is full of challenges, but it's also full of beauty. There's always a reason to wag your tail, no matter how hard things might seem at times. Whether it's the love of a family, the warmth of the sun, or the simple pleasure of a tasty treat (bacon, anyone?), life has so much to offer if we just stay open to it.

We don't always know what the future holds, but that's okay. Sometimes, the greatest adventures come from the unknown. As long as we keep moving forward—one paw in front of the other—and stay true to who we are, everything will work out.

I've learned that the journey isn't always easy, but it's always worth it. Whether you're human or dog, life will throw challenges your way, but if you face them with an open heart, you'll come out stronger and more fulfilled.

## A Final Thought on Happiness

You're going to realize one day that happiness was never about your job, your degree, or being in a relationship. It was never about following in the footsteps of others or trying to be like someone else. Happiness has always been about discovery—about listening to your heart and following it wherever it leads you.

It's about being kinder to yourself, embracing the person (or dog) you're becoming, and finding peace in the journey. One day, you'll understand that happiness was never in the hands of others—it was always within you.

So, be gentle with yourself. Celebrate the small victories. Savor the quiet moments. Love the ones around you deeply and freely. That's where true happiness lies—not in the world's expectations, but in the way you choose to live and love.

## A Promise to Keep Exploring

As I bring this story to a close, I want to thank you for being a part of my journey. Every adventure, every new friend, every moment of growth—it's all been worth it because I've had you along for the ride.

And this isn't the end. There are always new adventures on the horizon. Maybe next time I'll write about the best dog treats out there, or maybe I'll do something like my Dad does

with pizza and start rating them! Who knows? The possibilities are endless, and I'm excited to see where life takes me next.

But whatever comes next, remember this: we're all in this together. Whether you're human or dog, we're all walking this journey side by side, sniffing out the good things, embracing the challenges, and finding joy in the ride.

## You Are Always Loved!

So, until next time, friends, keep wagging your tails and enjoying the little things. Never forget that you are always loved, and no matter where life takes you, there's always happiness to be found if you just keep looking for it.

Woof! Or Meow… whatever that means!

# AUTHOR'S PERSPECTIVE
## *JOHN RINALDO*

When I set out to write Remi's Story, my goal wasn't just to share the adventures of a lovable, loyal dog. I wanted to shine a light on something close to my heart—adopting dogs and the profound impact they can have on our lives. Throughout Remi's journey, I aimed to showcase not only the joys but also the responsibilities that come with caring for a dog, particularly a rescue or an adopted pet.

Adopting a dog is more than just bringing home a new family member; it's about giving a second chance to a creature that often comes from challenging circumstances. Dogs like Remi, who have experienced separation from their original families or have lived in foster care, carry their own stories. When we adopt them, we become part of their healing, and they, in turn, become part of ours. Their loyalty, unconditional love, and ability to bring happiness into our lives are immeasurable, but it's important to remember that this bond requires care, patience, and responsibility.

Why Adoption?

There are millions of dogs waiting in shelters, hoping for a forever home. Many of these dogs are there through no fault of their own—perhaps their owners could no longer care for them, or they were abandoned. Adopting a dog not only gives them a second chance at a better life but also helps reduce overpopulation in shelters.

I wanted Remi's story to highlight that adopted dogs, regardless of their background, are not "less than" those bred for specific traits. They are just as capable of being loyal companions, support animals, or even skilled performers, as seen in Remi's journey. When you adopt, you're not only saving a life, but you're also gaining a lifelong friend who will love you unconditionally.

**The Responsibilities of Dog Ownership**

Owning a dog comes with a deep sense of responsibility. Through Remi's eyes, I wanted to illustrate the balance between the joy of having a dog and the commitment it requires. From training sessions with "Dad" to the emotional support Remi provides his family, every chapter reflects the mutual care needed to maintain a healthy, happy relationship with a pet.

• **Training:** As shown in Remi's story, consistent training is essential for a dog's safety and well-being. It strengthens the bond between dog and owner, provides mental stimulation, and helps the dog understand their role within the family.

• **Exercise and Health:** Dogs like Remi thrive on physical and mental activity. Regular walks, playtime, and challenges are crucial for keeping them fit and emotionally balanced. Owning a dog isn't just about feeding and housing them; it's about ensuring their overall well-being, which includes grooming, vet checkups, and maintaining a stimulating environment.

• **Love and Patience:** Many dogs, especially those who have been adopted, need time to adjust to their new surroundings. I hope Remi's experiences with change—moving to a new home, meeting new people—show the importance of patience and love in helping a dog transition into their new life.

**Bringing Awareness**

The purpose of Remi's Story is to bring awareness to the importance of adopting dogs and understanding the commitment it entails. It's easy to fall in love with the idea of having a dog but caring for one is a lifelong responsibility. I hope that through Remi's journey, readers can see that while it requires work, the reward is immeasurable.

Dogs are more than pets—they're companions who can bring us peace, joy, and love in ways we never expected. But to receive all of this, we need to be prepared to give them the care, love, and respect they deserve. By adopting, we're not only changing the life of a dog; we're changing our own in the process.

Through Remi's Story, I hope readers will be inspired to consider adopting a dog and understand the responsibilities that come with it. It's a journey of mutual care and growth, one that can bring incredible joy and fulfillment to both humans and dogs alike. And for those who already own dogs, I hope Remi's adventures serve as a reminder of the love and commitment we owe to these incredible creatures who give so much to us.

Adopting a dog isn't just about rescuing them—it's about discovering the depth of what they can bring into your life, and the ways they can help us grow, learn, and love in return.

Thank you for reading Remi's story! The next step in this journey is to bring these stories together into a book, so that others can share Remi's adventures with their family and friends. My hope is that Remi's experiences will inspire people to embrace the love and responsibility that comes with adopting and caring for dogs. Together, we can spread

the message of compassion, joy, and the transformative power of giving a dog a forever home. Stay tuned for the next chapter in Remi's journey!

~ John Rinaldo

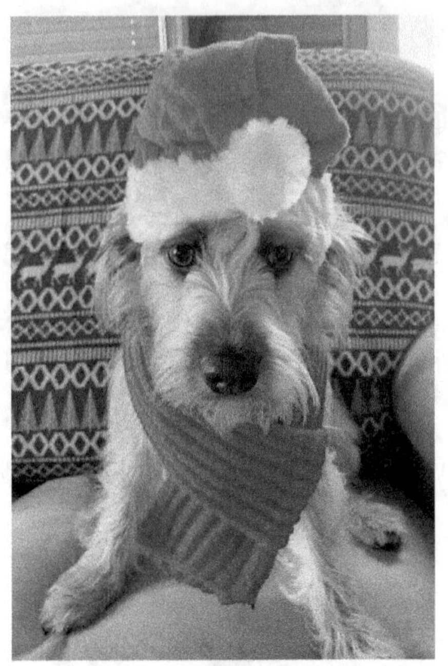

"Remi Playing Santa"

*"You know, a dog can snap you out of any kind of bad mood that you're in faster than you can think of."*

– Jill Abramson

# ABOUT THE AUTHOR

John V. Rinaldo is a multifaceted author whose works span a diverse range of topics, from personal anecdotes to uplifting narratives. His previous bestseller, Rediscovery of Vancouver (2023), captivated Canadian readers, and now, he invites you into the heartwarming world of Remi's Journey: *Tails of Love, Joy, and Hope*. The inspiration for this book comes directly from his own experience of raising Remi, his beloved dog, and the lessons learned along the way.

Through his writing, John extends a heartfelt invitation to readers to join him on a personal journey filled with stories that resonate deeply. His books are available on Amazon, where readers can discover narratives that inspire and engage.

John's storytelling goes beyond traditional books. Writing under the pen name Positive Pen, he uses Substack as a unique platform where readers can witness the raw, unedited development of his books. By sharing draft chapters and encouraging feedback, John offers his audience a chance to influence the final publication. This interactive writing process has become a hallmark of his work, making his books not only a personal creation but a collaborative effort between author and reader.

Through this approach, John V. Rinaldo has carved out a niche as a storyteller who masterfully blends personal experiences, inspiration, and positivity into narratives that speak to a wide audience. Whether you're reading his published books or following his creative journey on Substack, John's engaging and genuine writing encourages readers to embrace the adventure of life and find joy in everyday moments.

Don't miss the opportunity to follow John's inspirational musings and creative process on social media, and experience firsthand the evolution of his next great story.

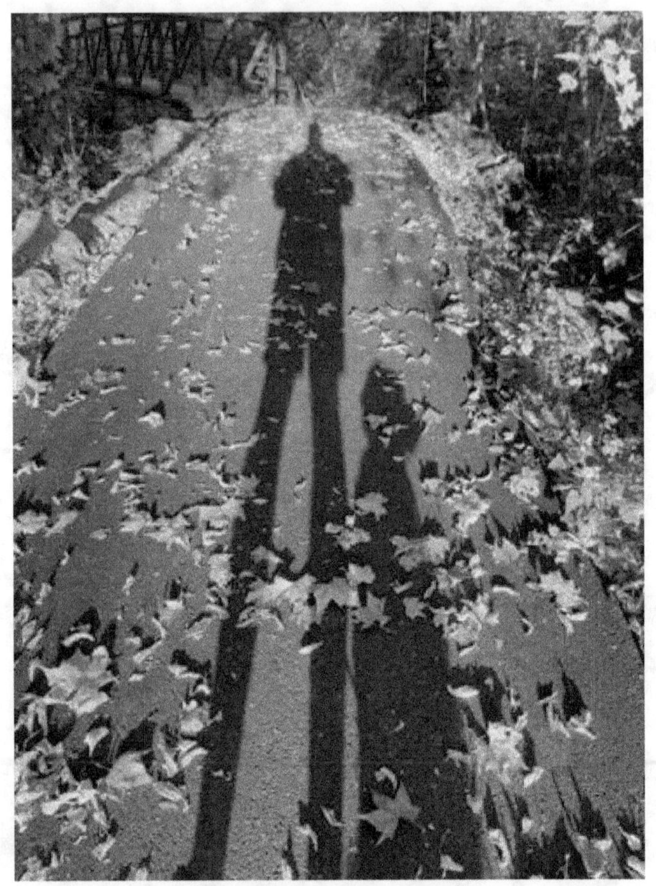



*"Before you get a dog, you can't quite imagine what living with one might be like; afterward, you can't imagine living any other way."*

– Caroline Knapp

# AUTHOR'S PUBLICANS

The following titles by John Rinaldo are available for purchase on Amazon or at www.RinaldoPartners.com:

1. **Surviving COVID-19:** *Being Alone Was the Best COVID-19 Medicine*
2. **The Bike Accident:** *Working Through the Low Valleys of Blessings*
3. **Eternal Whispers:** *A Love Story of Richelle and Matteo*
4. **Rediscovering Vancouver:** *A Journey of Memories and Natural Beauty*
5. **Remi's Journey:** *Tails of Love, Joy, and Hope*

To stay updated with John Rinaldo, also known as the *Positive Pen*, follow his Substack at rinaldoj.substack.com. There, he shares the inspirations behind his books and more, including:

1. **100 Inspirational Days**
2. **Rediscovering Vancouver**
3. **Daily Thoughts**
4. **Remembrance**
5. **Remi's Journey**

On Substack, John invites you on a unique storytelling journey. You'll get a behind-the-scenes look at his creative process, witnessing how his daily writings evolve into full-fledged books. It's an opportunity to engage with the origins of his stories and become part of the positive narrative he brings to life.

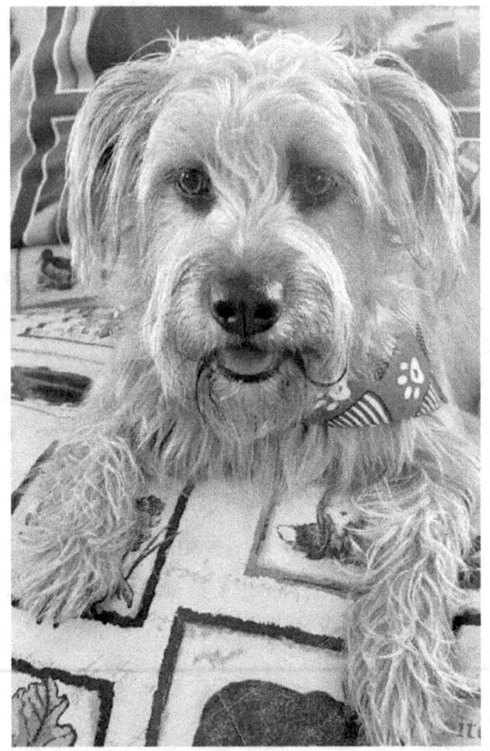

"REMI TIME"

*"A boy can learn a lot from a dog: obedience, loyalty, and the importance of turning around three times before lying down."*

– Robert Benchley

9 798340 049377